Glossary of abbreviations

ADAMTS-13: a disintegrin-like and metalloprotease with thrombospondin type 1 motif 13

ADP: adenosine diphosphate

APTT: activated partial thromboplastin time

cAMP: cyclic adenosine monophosphate

cGMP: cyclic guanosine monophosphate

CNS: central nervous system

DIC: disseminated intravascular coagulation

EACA: ε-aminocaproic acid

EDTA: ethylenediamine tetra-acetic acid

FDP: fibrin degradation product

Gp: glycoprotein

HELLP: hemolytic anemia with elevated liver enzymes and low platelet count

HHT: hereditary hemorrhagic telangiectasia

HIT: heparin-induced thrombocytopenia

HIV: human immunodeficiency virus

HLA: human leukocyte antigen

HUS: hemolytic uremic syndrome

ICAM: intercellular adhesion molecule

Ig: immunoglobulin

IL: interleukin

INR: international normalized ratio

ITP: immune thrombocytopenic purpura

LDH: lactic dehydrogenase

LMWH: low molecular weight heparin

MW: molecular weight

NAIT: neonatal alloimmune thrombocytopenia

NSAID: non-steroidal anti-inflammatory drug

PAI: plasminogen activator inhibitor

PFA: platelet function analyzer

PIH: pregnancy-induced hypertension

PT: prothrombin time

rapC: recombinant human activated protein C

TAFI: thrombin activatable fibrinolysis inhibitor

TF: tissue factor

TFPI: tissue factor pathway inhibitor

TGFβ: transforming growth factor β

TNFα: tumor necrosis factor α

tPA: tissue plasminogen activator

TTP: thrombotic thrombocytopenic purpura

VCAM: vascular cell adhesion molecule

vWD: von Willebrand's disease

vWF: von Willebrand factor

Introduction

Bleeding disorders have had a major impact on world history, beginning with injunctions about practicing ritual circumcision in individuals with a family history of bleeding, to the spread of hemophilia throughout the royal families of Europe by the descendants of Queen Victoria. Bleeding has also been a major cause of mortality after trauma and has dogged surgical procedures. Hemorrhage may be overt or extremely subtle, and may occur unexpectedly in association with a variety of illnesses.

This book begins by describing normal hemostatic mechanisms and suggests how alterations in coagulation may be suspected from the clinical history and examination, and confirmed by laboratory testing. Many bleeding disorders are due to vascular anomalies and vasculitis, and hereditary hemorrhagic telangiectasia (HHT) and Henoch–Schönlein purpura, for example, are discussed in detail. Platelet function disturbances may also promote bleeding, and may be congenital or acquired secondary to exposure to aspirin and other platelet inhibitors used to prevent thrombosis. A simple algorithm is presented to aid the differential diagnosis of thrombocytopenia, and the appropriate use of platelet transfusions and other hemostatic agents is discussed.

The diagnosis and treatment of hemophilia, von Willebrand's disease (vWD) and other inherited coagulopathies is outlined, and currently available therapeutic products described. Advice on the approach to bleeding that often complicates liver and kidney disorders, which may be multifactorial, is also presented. Bleeding disorders during pregnancy constitute a risk to mother and fetus, and must be recognized promptly and treated effectively. Perioperative bleeding is due to a failure of local hemostasis, or to a variety of systemic causes, including hemodilution, vitamin K deficiency and drugs. Disseminated intravascular coagulation (DIC) complicates acute sepsis, obstetric conditions and malignant disease, and requires accurate diagnosis and appropriate management. Finally, anticoagulants may be pathological proteins that arise in a patient and alter coagulation, or therapeutic agents that cause bleeding as an important adverse effect. A wide-ranging discussion of the management of hemorrhage associated with the most commonly used antithrombotic agents completes the text.

When a physician encounters a bleeding patient, diagnostic and therapeutic steps need to be taken rapidly. It is our hope that *Fast Facts – Bleeding Disorders*, prepared so that information about bleeding disorders is readily accessible, will improve patient management and outcomes.

Normal hemostasis

In health, hemostasis ensures that the blood remains fluid and contained within the vasculature. If a vessel wall is damaged, a number of mechanisms are activated promptly to limit bleeding by a complex series of interrelated reactions involving endothelial cells, plasma coagulation factors, platelets and fibrinolytic proteins. The activities of these components are finely balanced between keeping the blood fluid and preventing excessive activation of the procoagulatory components leading to intravascular thrombosis.

It is helpful to consider the hemostatic process as three distinct phases.

- Primary hemostasis occurs after damage to the vessel wall, and involves vasoconstriction and adhesion of platelets in a monolayer on exposed subendothelial fibrils. Subsequently, further platelets aggregate to form a platelet plug, which stems the flow of blood.
- Secondary hemostasis involves activation of the coagulation system, leading to the generation of fibrin strands, which are laid down between platelets and reinforce the platelet plug.
- Fibrinolysis entails activation of fibrin-bound plasminogen, resulting in clot lysis. Lysis is modulated by inhibitors of fibrinolysis activated by thrombin or released by platelets.

In reality, these processes tend to merge, with the activated platelet and endothelial cell membranes providing the foundation on which the clotting factors can become activated, and fibrin formed and lysed.

Endothelial cells
Blood vessels are lined with endothelial cells, which promote hemostasis and keep the blood fluid by preventing excessive deposition of fibrin through the synthesis and secretion of various antithrombotic agents (Table 1.1). Endothelial cells also synthesize proteins that directly promote hemostasis. Von Willebrand factor (vWF) is synthesized by both endothelial cells and megakaryocytes (leading to its presence in platelet α-granules). When the endothelium is damaged, the

TABLE 1.1

Role of endothelial cells in hemostasis

Factors in endothelial cells	Activity
Procoagulant (prothrombotic)	
Tissue factor	Initiates coagulation cascade
von Willebrand factor	Promotes adhesion of platelets
Factors V and VIII	Essential cofactors for coagulation
Plasminogen activator inhibitor-1	Inhibits fibrinolysis
Cytokines (e.g. interleukin-6)	Proinflammatory
Cellular adhesion molecules (e.g. intercellular adhesion molecule, vascular cell adhesion molecule)	Promotes adhesion of neutrophils
Anticoagulant (antithrombotic)	
Tissue factor pathway inhibitor	Inhibits initiation of coagulation
Prostacyclin	Platelet inhibitor and vasodilator
Nitric oxide	Platelet inhibitor and vasodilator
Endothelin-1	Platelet inhibitor and vasoconstrictor
Thrombomodulin and protein C receptor	Redirects thrombin activity towards activating protein C/S anticoagulant system
Tissue plasminogen activator	Promotes fibrinolysis
Heparan sulfate	Binds and enhances the activity of antithrombin

subendothelial vessel wall components are exposed, and vWF promotes adhesion of circulating platelets to the exposed microfibrils and collagen. Stimulation of the endothelium by thrombin, following activation of the coagulation cascade, or by cytokines, such as tumor necrosis factor α (TNFα), promotes the synthesis and expression of tissue factor (TF) on the cell surface. This complexes with circulating plasma coagulation factor VII to form TF–VIIa which initiates the coagulation cascade. Stimulated endothelial cells synthesize other proteins that promote hemostasis, such as plasminogen activator inhibitor (PAI)-1, as well as cell adhesion molecules (e.g. vascular cell adhesion molecule 1, VCAM1), which promote accumulation of white cells. Endothelial cells also secrete: heparan sulfate, which inhibits activated clotting factors; prostacyclin and nitric oxide, which inhibit platelet aggregation and induce vasodilatation; and tissue plasminogen activator (tPA), which promotes the dissolution of fibrin that is deposited within the vasculature. This prevents excessive fibrin deposition and thrombosis.

Platelets

Each bone marrow megakaryocyte produces approximately 1000–2000 platelets, which remain in the circulation for about 10 days. These highly specialized anucleate cells (Figure 1.1) take part in a series of complex reactions to prevent blood loss. On escaping from a damaged vessel at high shear rates, the platelet adheres, via its surface glycoprotein (Gp) 1b-IX-V, to vWF and collagen in the subendothelial vessel wall. This activates the platelet, causing exposure of the fibrinogen receptor Gp IIb/IIIa. Other important receptors are P2Y1 and P2Y12 for adenosine diphosphate (ADP), and thrombin and thromboxane receptors. Binding of these ligands to their receptors induces platelet activation and aggregation. Hemostatic proteins, such as vWF and fibrinogen, are released from the α-granules and promote

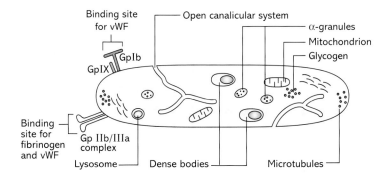

Figure 1.1 The structure of a platelet. vWF, von Willebrand factor; Gp, glycoprotein.

cross-linking between platelets to help the development of a platelet plug to stem the hemorrhage. In addition, ADP and serotonin (5-hydroxytryptamine) are released from platelet dense granules, and promote further aggregation of platelets and vasoconstriction of the blood vessel. Activation of the platelet membranes also provides receptors for other plasma coagulation factors (e.g. prothrombin and factors V, X and XI). Thus, the activated platelet membrane provides a surface on which the components of coagulation can gather very rapidly, leading to the development of a 'fibrin-reinforced' stable platelet plug.

Coagulation system

The coagulation factors are a series of plasma proteins synthesized in the liver which, when activated, lead via a sequence of complex reactions to the deposition of fibrin. Although originally conceived as a simple cascade, it is now viewed as an interrelated network of reactions, initiated by TF expressed by the endothelium, and supported by the accumulation of the components of coagulation on specific receptors on the activated platelet membrane (Figure 1.2). During the *initiation phase* of coagulation, the endothelial cell is activated, as outlined above, leading to the expression of TF on the cell surface. This is a receptor for circulating factor VII, which forms the complex TF–VIIa and initiates the *amplification phase* of the coagulation cascade by activating factor X to Xa, and to a lesser extent factor IX to IXa, on the platelet surface. Factor Xa, along with factor V (which it activates to Va), catalyzes the formation of a small amount of thrombin from its precursor prothrombin. This thrombin initiates a *propagation phase* in which several positive feedback reactions result in the generation of much larger amounts of thrombin. One of the important feedback reactions by thrombin is the activation of factor XI to XIa. Factor XIa binds to platelet Gp Ib and activates factor IX. Activated factor IX, with factor VIII as a cofactor, activates factor X. Factor Xa, along with activated factor V, converts prothrombin, which has bound to platelet Gp IIb/IIIa, to thrombin. The explosive generation of further thrombin converts large amounts of fibrinogen to fibrin. This is stabilized by cross-linking by factor XIIIa, which is

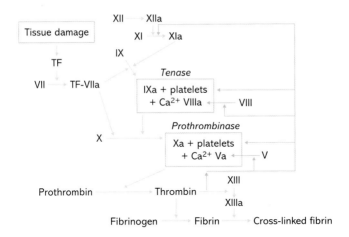

Figure 1.2 Coagulation system. Clotting is initiated by tissue factor (TF) expressed on damaged or activated cells. The enzyme complexes tenase and prothrobinase form on the platelet surface. The blue lines represent the positive feedback effects (propagation) of small amounts of thrombin, which greatly enhance the activity of the coagulation network and result in large amounts of thrombin and thus fibrin (clot) formation. The clotting factors are represented by Roman numerals alone.

activated from factor XIII by thrombin. Thrombin is also a potent activator of platelets, which provide an enhanced catalytic surface on which further coagulation is promoted. The activated platelets release hemostatic factors (e.g. fibrinogen and vWF) that recruit further platelets into the aggregates (see page 10).

As well as having a pivotal role in promoting coagulation, thrombin is an important regulator of fibrinolysis (see page 12).

Inhibitors of coagulation. The plasma contains a series of proteins that inhibit activated procoagulant enzymes and prevent excessive intravascular coagulation. Raised levels of these inhibitors are not associated with a bleeding state, but a reduced concentration may predispose to thrombosis.

Antithrombin is a potent and clinically very important inhibitor of thrombin, factors Xa and XIa, and the TF–VIIa complex. It limits the

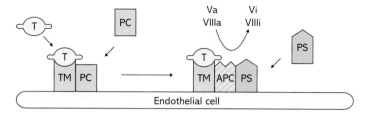

Figure 1.3 Protein C pathway. Thrombin (T), generated by the coagulation network, binds to thrombomodulin (TM) on the endothelial cell membrane. Protein C (PC) binds to the endothelial protein C receptor and is converted by thrombomodulin-bound thrombin to activated protein C (APC). When the plasma cofactor protein S (PS) binds to activated protein C, it can inactivate activated factor V (Va) and VIII (VIIIa) to inactive molecules Vi and VIIIi. Thus a deficiency in the protein C/S pathway leads to persistence of Va and VIIIa, which predispose to thrombosis and may modify the severity of inherited bleeding disorders.

overall activation of the coagulation mechanism, preventing excessive fibrin deposition and thrombosis.

Protein C. The protein C pathway is a further mechanism by which intravascular coagulation is limited (Figure 1.3). This pathway is initiated by thrombin when it binds to thrombomodulin on the endothelial surface and activates protein C bound to its receptor on the cell membrane. Activated protein C, along with its cofactor, free protein S, inactivates the activated coagulation proteins Va and VIIIa by proteolysis. Protein Z binds to the Z-protease inhibitor and the complex inactivates factor Xa.

Tissue factor pathway inhibitor (TFPI) binds factor Xa, forming a complex that rapidly inhibits the TF–VIIa complex.

Inhibitor deficiency. A deficiency of antithrombin or proteins C or S predisposes to venous thromboembolism, because the overall activity of the coagulation system is insufficiently inhibited. The importance of protein Z and TFPI in hemostasis is still being evaluated.

Fibrinolysis

Small amounts of fibrin are constantly being deposited within the vasculature and are removed by the fibrinolytic system (Figure 1.4).

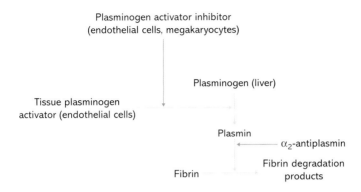

Figure 1.4 Fibrinolysis. The red lines represent inhibitors.

This pathway consists of an initiator, tPA, which is synthesized and released from endothelial cells. tPA converts its substrate plasminogen (which is bound within the clot to fibrin) to plasmin, which in turn lyses intravascular fibrin to soluble fibrin degradation products (FDPs). FDPs consist of fragments of cross-linked fibrin known as D-dimers, which can be measured in the laboratory and reflect the amount of fibrin degradation. The small amounts of plasmin escaping from the clot are neutralized by circulating antiplasmin.

Inhibitors of fibrinolysis. Fibrinolysis is also inhibited by specific inhibitors.

Plasminogen activator inhibitor-1, which is synthesized by endothelial cells, and antiplasmin inhibit tPA and plasmin, respectively. Raised levels of PAI-1 are associated with atheroma, though it is unclear whether a high plasma level predisposes to, or is a consequence of, atherothrombosis. Raised antiplasmin levels do not appear to predispose to thrombosis, though low levels occasionally lead to a bleeding state because of the unopposed action of plasmin.

Plasminogen activator inhibitor-2 is synthesized by the placenta and is an important inhibitor of tPA, especially at the end of pregnancy.

Thrombin activatable fibrinolytic inhibitor (TAFI) is a recently described fibrinolytic inhibitor activated by thrombin. TAFI is a carboxypeptidase that cleaves lysine from fibrin, preventing plasminogen binding to fibrin. When thrombin generation is defective, as in hemophilia, impaired activation of TAFI may result in enhanced fibrinolysis and bleeding.

Key points – hemostasis

- The immediate arrest of hemorrhage depends on vasoconstriction along with the adhesion and aggregation of platelets at the site of vessel injury.
- The coagulation system is activated by tissue factor expression. This binds and converts factor VII to VIIa, which initiates a catalytic series of reactions leading to the rapid generation of small amounts of thrombin.
- The initial trace concentrations of thrombin trigger the explosive generation of a much larger quantity of thrombin by activating factors XI, VIII and V in a positive feedback loop.
- Thrombin further promotes the stability of the platelet–fibrin hemostatic plug by activating more platelets, factor XIII (cross-linking fibrin strands) and thrombin activatable fibrinolytic inhibitor.

Key references

Butenas S, Mann KG. Blood coagulation. *Biochemistry* 2002;67:3–12.

Colman RW, Hirsh J, Marder VJ, Clowes AW. Overview of coagulation, fibrinolysis and their regulation. In: Colman RW, Hirsh J, Marder VJ et al., eds. *Haemostasis and Thrombosis*. 4th edn. London: Lippincott, Williams and Wilkins, 2000:17–20.

Heemskerk JW, Bevers EM, Lindhout T. Platelet activation and blood coagulation. *Thromb Haemost* 2002;88:186–93.

Hoffman M, Monroe DM. A cell-based model of hemostasis. *Thromb Haemost* 2001;85:958–65.

Hutton RA, Laffan MA, Tuddenham EGD. Normal haemostasis. In: Hoffbrand AV, Lewis SM, Tuddenham EGD, eds. *Postgraduate Haematology*. 4th edn. Oxford: Heinemann, 1998:550–80.

Mann KG, Butenas S, Brummell K. The dynamics of thrombin generation. *Arterioscler Thromb Vasc Biol* 2003;23:17–25.

For most patients, assessment of the hemostatic system comprises:
• a careful and full clinical history and examination
• appropriate laboratory investigations.
It is important to try to assess the likelihood of the patient having a bleeding disorder from the history, as this will determine the extent of the subsequent investigations. For example, a patient who has bled on multiple occasions from different anatomic sites merits more extensive laboratory investigation than an individual who has bled repeatedly from a single site (e.g. a peptic ulcer). The history should also suggest whether there is a disorder of primary hemostasis (i.e. a platelet abnormality or vWD) or an abnormality of secondary hemostasis (e.g. hemophilia).

History

A full general medical history and examination should be undertaken, and the bleeding symptoms assessed in the context of the patient's overall health and lifestyle.

Site of bleed. Failure of the primary hemostatic system results in bruising, purpura, prolonged bleeding from superficial cuts, epistaxis, gastrointestinal bleeding and menorrhagia, and is usually due to a platelet abnormality or vWD. Disorders of secondary hemostasis, caused by abnormalities in the propagation of coagulation reactions, lead to hemarthroses and muscle hematoma. Recurrent bleeding from a single anatomic site (e.g. epistaxis from a single nostril) is most likely to result from a structural abnormality rather than a defect in the hemostatic system, whereas bleeding at many different sites suggests a systemic hemostatic defect.

Duration of bleeding. Bleeding symptoms occurring over a long period of time suggest a life-long congenital bleeding disorder, while those of recent origin may be more in keeping with an acquired disorder (e.g. liver disease). Difficulties may arise in individuals with mild congenital bleeding disorders, who often only bleed after surgery and who may remain undiagnosed until adulthood, especially now that circumcision, tonsillectomy and dental extractions are performed less often in childhood.

Precipitating cause. Bleeding that arises spontaneously reflects the presence of a more severe bleeding state than hemorrhage which occurs only after surgery or trauma.

Surgery. It is important to ask about all operations, especially dental extractions, tonsillectomy and circumcision, as these are particularly severe stresses to the hemostatic system. It can also be helpful to know when the bleeding occurred after surgery. Bleeding that starts immediately indicates a platelet abnormality or vWD. On the other hand, hemorrhage that is delayed for several hours after surgery suggests a clotting factor disorder; the delay occurs because the primary platelet plug disintegrates following inadequate consolidation with fibrin strands.

Family history. A positive family history of bleeding disorder can be helpful in directing investigations (e.g. hemophilia). However, the absence of a family history does not exclude a heritable condition: new mutations are present in about one-third of hemophiliacs; and, in those with mild bleeding disorders, other affected relatives may not have been diagnosed.

Systemic illness. Medical conditions that predispose to bleeding, such as renal or liver failure, paraproteinemia and collagenoses, should be considered. In acutely ill patients, there are often multiple reasons for bleeding (e.g. septicemia, uremia and the effect of drugs).

Drugs. It is essential to obtain a full drug history, as nearly all medicines can inhibit the bone marrow with resultant thrombocytopenia, and most interact with oral anticoagulants. Non-steroidal anti-inflammatory drugs (NSAIDs) are in widespread use as analgesics and many inhibit platelet function. Aspirin is widely used as an antithrombotic; it induces a mild predisposition to bleeding in most individuals and this may unmask an underlying lifelong mild bleeding disorder. It is important to inquire specifically about oral anticoagulant therapy and, in hospitalized patients, the use of unfractionated or low molecular weight heparin (LMWH) as prophylaxis against venous thromboembolism.

Examination

Superficial examination. The skin should be examined carefully for bruising and purpura. The mouth may contain small hemorrhagic bullae. A single large bullus on the palate is characteristic of angina bullosa hemorrhagica, a condition of unknown etiology that is not associated with an underlying bleeding disorder. Bruising around the head and neck should raise the possibility of trauma and, in children, consideration must be given to the possibility of non-accidental injury. Telangiectasia on the lips, tongue or fingertips is seen in HHT. The large joints should be examined for acute hemarthroses or evidence of previous damage from bleeds, as may be found in hemophilia. Scars over the elbows and knees are a feature of factor XIII deficiency. Turner's sign appears as bruising over the flanks due to tracking of blood arising from either the peritoneum or retroperitoneum along the subcutaneous tissue. Cullen's sign appears as periumbilical ecchymoses due to tracking of blood along the falciform ligament; it occurs in hemorrhagic pancreatitis, liver tumor, splenic rupture, ruptured ectopic pregnancy, leaking aortic aneurysm and retroperitoneal hemorrhage.

General examination. A full examination should be carried out to look for evidence of other disorders, such as the stigmata of liver disease, evidence of malignancy, lymphadenopathy and hepatosplenomegaly. If severe thrombocytopenia is suspected, the optic fundi should be examined for evidence of intraocular bleeding. Furthermore, in a drowsy or comatose patient, it is important to consider the possibility of an intracranial bleed.

Local lesion. Attempts should be made to visualize all bleeding points by endoscopy (Figure 2.1), ultrasound, computerized tomography (CT)

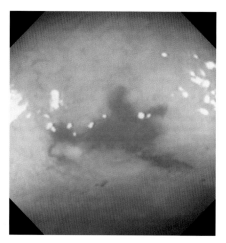

Figure 2.1 Bleeding telangiectasia as seen on endoscopy. Reprinted with permission from Elsevier (Hodgson H. *Lancet* 2002;359:1630).

or magnetic resonance imaging (MRI). In addition to assessing the severity of bleeding, this may also establish whether an underlying structural abnormality is present.

Investigations

Once a full history and the results of the physical examination have been obtained, it should be possible to assess whether the patient has a disorder of primary or secondary hemostasis, and its severity. The extent of the investigations will depend on the likelihood of the patient having a bleeding disorder. It is customary to begin with a full blood count, blood film and coagulation screen. If the history is not particularly suggestive of a bleeding disorder, these investigations may be sufficient. On the other hand, if the patient has a very convincing history but normal screening tests, it would be appropriate to consider measuring levels of the individual coagulation factors, usually beginning with factor VIII and vWF, as hemophilia A and vWD are the most common congenital bleeding disorders.

Full blood count. A full blood count and examination of the blood film may reveal evidence of a previously unsuspected disorder, such as leukemia or liver disease. The platelet count (Table 2.1) and the

TABLE 2.1

Screening investigations to detect a hemorrhagic state

Investigation	Components assessed	Conditions in which test is abnormal
Platelet count	Platelets	Congenital and acquired platelet disorders (see Table 4.2, page 37)
Bleeding time	Platelet function von Willebrand factor	Functional platelet disorder von Willebrand's disease
Prothrombin time	Factors II, V, VII and X	Warfarin Liver disease Congenital factor deficiencies DIC Lupus inhibitor
Activated partial thromboplastin time	Factors V, VIII, IX, X, XI and XII	Unfractionated heparin DIC Congenital factor deficiencies Anti-factor VIII antibody Lupus inhibitor
Fibrinogen concentration	Fibrinogen	DIC Congenital hypofibrinogenemia Severe liver disease
Fibrin degradation products	Lysis of fibrin	DIC

DIC, disseminated intravascular coagulation.

morphology of these cells are important. Large platelets are characteristic of some of the hereditary platelet disorders (Figure 2.2), and are also found in primary thrombocythemia and other myeloproliferative conditions.

Bleeding time. If the platelet count is above $50 \times 10^9/L$ and a platelet function disorder or vWD is suspected, a bleeding time test may be appropriate (Figure 2.3).

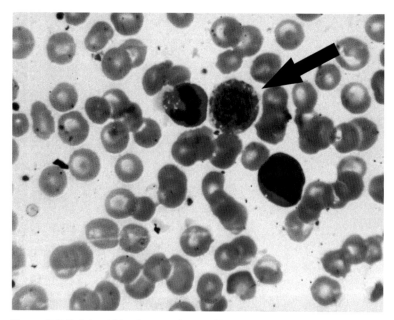

Figure 2.2 Peripheral blood smear showing May–Hegglin disorder with giant platelets and a Döhle body in a leukocyte (arrow). (Wright's stain × 400.)

Coagulation screen. A coagulation screen involves measurement of activated partial thromboplastin time (APTT), prothrombin time (PT) and fibrinogen concentration. The APTT clotting test is initiated by activation of factor XII and is therefore prolonged when deficiencies of factors XII, XI, IX, VIII, X and V are present. It should be noted that factor XII deficiency is not associated with a predisposition to bleeding. The PT is performed by adding TF to plasma and is prolonged when levels of factors II, VII, X and V are low. These screening tests are insensitive to small reductions in the levels of clotting factors; therefore, if the clinical possibility of a mild bleeding disorder is high, the level of individual factors must be measured.

If the platelet count and morphology are normal, but a platelet function disorder is suspected, further investigation is necessary. Platelet aggregation can be measured in response to ADP, epinephrine and collagen, and the concentration of ADP in the platelet dense granules can be quantitated.

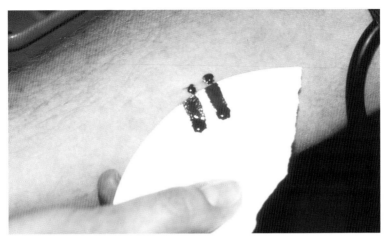

Figure 2.3 To determine the bleeding time, two standardized, superficial incisions of 0.5 cm in length and 1 mm in depth are made along the long axis of the forearm, below the antecubital crease. To stress the hemostatic mechanism, venous pressure is increased using a sphygmomanometer cuff on the upper arm inflated to 40 mmHg. The incisions are dabbed with filter paper every 30 seconds and the time taken until bleeding stops is measured; the normal time is less than 8 minutes.

Key points – assessment of bleeding symptoms

- A full and detailed history of personal and family bleeding symptoms often indicates the nature and severity of a potential bleeding diathesis.
- All current and recent drugs should be reviewed as possible causes of a bleeding state.
- Specific inquiry should be made about oral anticoagulant or other antithrombotic therapy (e.g. aspirin).
- Defects of primary hemostasis (i.e. platelet disorders and von Willebrand's disease) present with mucosal bleeding (e.g. epistaxis, gastrointestinal hemorrhage and menorrhagia).
- Defects of secondary hemostasis (i.e. coagulation disorders such as hemophilia) usually present with hemarthroses and muscle hematoma.

Key references

Chee YL, Greaves M. Role of coagulation testing in predicting bleeding risk. *Hematology J* 2003;4:373–8.

Greaves M, Preston FE. Approach to the bleeding patient. In: Colman RW, Hirsh J, Marder VJ, Clowes AW, George JN, eds. *Haemostasis and Thrombosis*. 4th edn. London: Lippincot, Williams and Wilkins, 2000;783–94.

Hereditary hemorrhagic telangiectasia

Hereditary hemorrhagic telangiectasia (HHT) is classified as a vascular purpura. It is inherited as an autosomal disorder. The most common mutations are in the endoglin gene (*ENG*) at position 9q33-q34. The product of *ENG* is a cellular receptor for transforming growth factor β (TGFβ), which also binds to TGFβ receptors on endothelial and smooth muscle cells, thereby regulating signaling by this cytokine. Because TGFβ signaling is essential for vascular growth and development, defects in endoglin lead to the vascular malformations typical of HHT. The second group of mutations are in the gene for activin-receptor-like kinase 1, a protein that forms complexes with endoglin and TGFβ on the surface of endothelial cells.

Clinical features. Individuals with HHT have vascular malformations in the skin, nasal membranes, lung, brain, eye, liver and gastrointestinal tract. These telangiectasias typically have small feeding vessels and blanch with pressure. They are often found on the hands and fingertips (Figure 3.1); telangiectasias that occur in pregnancy and liver disease are usually located on the face and chest.

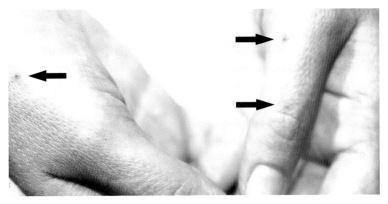

Figure 3.1 Telangiectasias on the fingers of a patient with hereditary hemorrhagic telangiectasia.

Two main pathological features characterize telangiectasias: they bleed freely when traumatized, and they may serve as arteriovenous conduits. Recurrent bleeding from the nose should raise suspicion of HHT and prompt a careful inspection of the nasal mucosa. Bleeding from the gastrointestinal tract may be quite subtle and manifest only by the development of iron deficiency anemia. Stool examination may reveal occult blood, but bleeding may be intermittent. The diagnosis is usually established by performing upper and lower endoscopy of the gastrointestinal tract and directly visualizing the telangiectasias. Lesions in the lung are often multiple, are generally in the lower lobes, and may enlarge and rupture, resulting in pulmonary hemorrhage. The significant shunting of blood through arteriovenous fistulas is a major concern, leading to cyanosis and paradoxical emboli. Brain abscesses may also occur.

HHT may also affect the eyes. Conjunctival lesions are commonly observed, and telangiectasias in the retina may bleed and provoke retinal detachment. Liver involvement occurs in up to one-third of patients with HHT. The presence of hepatic vascular malformations promotes a hyperdynamic circulation and high-output cardiac failure. Portal hypertension and biliary tract disease have also been reported. Portosystemic encephalopathy may develop if the toxic products of blood shed into the gut, or any medications administered, are shunted past the liver into the systemic circulation.

Management. A variety of treatments have been proposed for HHT, but the merits of each need to be carefully assessed for every individual patient. Patients readily become discouraged and depressed, but a hopeful, optimistic attitude should be maintained because of the many research advances that are being made and the potential for effective clinical applications in the near future.

Iron replacement therapy. Recurrent episodes of nosebleeding or gastrointestinal hemorrhage result in severe iron deficiency anemia requiring lifelong iron replacement therapy either orally or, occasionally, by regular intravenous infusions.

Measures to control bleeding are also necessary. HHT lesions are
associated with prominent fibrinolytic activity and therefore

ε-aminocaproic acid (EACA) or tranexamic acid may be indicated (see Chapter 5).

Hormonal therapy has been helpful in some patients with HHT. Oral estrogens containing norethisterone have been widely used, but may have intolerable side effects. Other steroids, including danazol and tamoxifen, have been employed as well as other compounds, such as soy products containing phytoestrogen and genistein, which interferes with the TGFβ pathway. There is, however, no single recommended treatment and none has been subjected to a randomized clinical trial.

Laser therapy or electrocautery has been a mainstay of treatment of mucosal telangiectasias in the nose or gastrointestinal mucosa. However, the benefit is often transitory, because bleeding recurs when the necrotic tissue sloughs. Giving an antifibrinolytic agent in conjunction with cautery may help obviate this problem. Most often, the telangiectasias are so numerous that it is difficult to identify which lesion is bleeding, and so a hit-or-miss strategy is employed in the hope that the culprit vessels will be obliterated. Arteriovenous fistulas and vascular malformations are usually managed by embolic therapy, surgical resection or radiosurgery.

Local measures should not be ignored in the management of HHT. Humidification, saline nasal spray and avoidance of nasal trauma may help prevent bleeding. Nasal packs are often inserted to control hemorrhage, but if left in place too long may damage the nasal mucosa and lead to recurrent bleeding. Septal dermoplasty is often of only temporary benefit as new telangiectatic lesions may form in the treated skin. Ultimately, many patients have vessels ligated and extensive amounts of tissue excised, but still continue to bleed. Therefore, treatment should be conservative and various agents prescribed until one is found to be effective.

Scurvy

Scurvy is a manifestation of vitamin C deficiency characterized by bleeding gums, perifollicular hemorrhages (Figure 3.2) and large ecchymoses on the buttocks and thighs. Although most patients have a long history of alcohol abuse and poor diet, a recent report described scurvy in a 6-year-old autistic boy who subsisted mainly on milk and

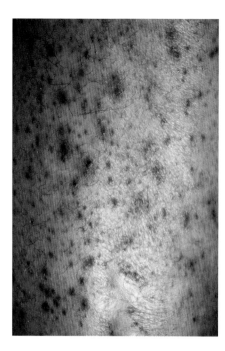

Figure 3.2 Perifollicular hemorrhages in a patient with scurvy.

cookies. In a unique study of five men on a diet lacking ascorbic acid, keratoconjunctivitis sicca, xerostomia and hyperkeratosis developed after 3–4 months without vitamin C. Mouth bleeding, perifollicular hemorrhages, dental decay and breakdown of dental restorations also occurred. Thus, the main diagnostic points are signs of poor nutrition, evidence of serious bleeding and normal laboratory screening tests for coagulation disorders. The response to therapy with vitamin C is dramatic; gum bleeding and ecchymoses subside within hours.

Henoch–Schönlein purpura

Henoch–Schönlein purpura is a form of immune vasculitis affecting venules in the skin, joints, intestinal mucosa and kidney. Deposits of immune complexes containing immunoglobulin (Ig) A can be identified in the circulation and in the walls of inflamed vessels. The cause of the condition is unknown, but cases have been described after exposure to aspirin, enalapril and carbidopa/levodopa. While children between the ages of 4 and 6 years are most commonly affected, the disease occasionally appears in adults. It has recently been reported that the annual incidence is 20.4/100 000. The clinical manifestations include vasculitic skin lesions and cutaneous ulcers (Figure 3.3), abdominal pain, arthopathy predominantly of the large joints and nephritis. Renal involvement is characterized by a crescentic proliferative glomerulonephritis. In a series of 20 patients, 7 (35%) who experienced severe Henoch–Schönlein purpura in childhood progressed to renal impairment in adulthood. In addition, women with a history of even mild renal symptoms were at risk of hypertension or proteinuria during pregnancy. Although some have urged merging Henoch–Schönlein purpura into the category of cutaneous vasculitis (palpable purpura), it appears that there are sufficient characteristic features (the IgA deposits, and the involvement of joints, intestinal mucosa and kidney) and risk of late renal sequelae to justify considering it as a specific entity. Once the diagnosis is established, usually by biopsy of skin or renal lesions, steroid therapy is initiated. However, as noted above, patients may progress to renal failure despite this treatment.

Mixed cryoglobulinemia

Occasionally, patients with hepatitis C infection develop circulating monoclonal IgM rheumatoid factor, which precipitates with polyclonal IgG at low temperature. Deposits of these immune complexes in skin

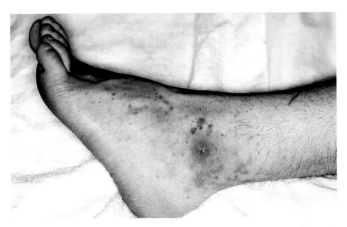

Figure 3.3 Vasculitic lesions and leg ulcer in a patient with Henoch–Schönlein purpura.

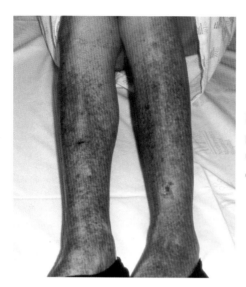

Figure 3.4 Vasculitis, pigmentation and shallow leg ulcers in a patient with mixed cryoglobulinemia.

venules, typically in the lower legs, result in extensive purpura (Figure 3.4). About 75% of patients have polyarthropathy and 50% develop renal involvement, usually glomerulonephritis. The diagnosis is suspected by observing purpura in the lower extremities, a skin biopsy showing hyaline deposits in the venules and cryoglobulin in serum stored at 4°C overnight. At this stage, serological tests for hepatitis C antibody or examination of the serum for the presence of hepatitis C RNA are indicated. Treatment with pegylated interferon and ribavirin may clear the hepatitis C viremia and lead to resolution of the mixed cryoglobulinemia.

Amyloid purpura

Deposition of amyloid in blood vessels markedly increases their fragility. Minor trauma, such as sneezing or putting the head in a dependent position, will cause small vessels to rupture and result in skin hemorrhage (Figure 3.5). Patients with amyloidosis may also come to medical attention as a result of proteinuria. If the diagnosis is not suspected and a renal biopsy is performed, there may be extensive retroperitoneal bleeding. A simple fat pad aspiration biopsy, stained with Congo red, may show the characteristic apple-green birefringence of amyloid material and establish the diagnosis. In addition to fragile

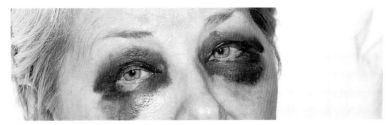

Figure 3.5 Raccoon eyes in a patient with amyloidosis.

blood vessels, patients with amyloidosis may have an acquired factor X deficiency due to binding of factor X to amyloid fibrils. Furthermore, patients with amyloidosis associated with multiple myeloma may have thrombocytopenia and other abnormalities of hemostasis. Thus, the management of this disorder may be quite complex. In one patient with factor X deficiency, recombinant human factor VIIa provided effective hemostasis for a major surgical procedure.

A different form of amyloid is found in the brain of patients with Alzheimer's disease, where it appears in plaques and in the walls of blood vessels. In an attempt to slow the progression of the disease, some patients were immunized with β-amyloid peptide. Unfortunately, this led to an increase in cerebral microhemorrhages associated with amyloid-laden vessels; this phenomenon has been reproduced in a mouse model of Alzheimer's disease. The amyloid-laden vessels may be more sensitive to the inflammatory reaction accompanying the immunologic attack on the vascular amyloid. The presence of amyloid in cerebral vessels (found in 10% of those over 65 years of age and in 80% of Alzheimer's patients) may also provide an explanation for the relatively high incidence of cerebral hemorrhage when these patients are treated with tPA.

Key points – vascular purpuras

• Individuals with recurrent nosebleeds and a family history of epistaxis should be carefully evaluated for hereditary hemorrhagic telangiectasia.

• Henoch–Schönlein purpura occurring in childhood may lead to complications in pregnancy and renal failure in adulthood.

• Palpable purpura, renal disease, polyarthropathy and cryoglobulinemia are usually associated with hepatitis C infection.

Key references

Boggio L, Green D.
Recombinant human factor VIIa
in the management of amyloid-
associated factor X deficiency.
Br J Haematol 2001;112:1074–5.

Bolton-Maggs PH, Pasi KJ.
Haemophilias A and B. *Lancet*
2003;361:1801–9.

Fornasieri A, D'Amico G.
Type II mixed cryoglobulinaemia,
hepatitis C virus infection, and
glomerulonephritis. *Nephrol Dial
Transplant* 1996;11(suppl 4):25–30.

Fuchizaki U, Miyamori H,
Kitagawa S et al. Hereditary
haemorrhagic telangectasia
(Rendu–Osler–Weber disease).
Lancet 2003;362:1490.

Garcia-Tsao G, Korzenik JR,
Young L et al. Liver disease in
patients with hereditary hemorrhagic
telangiectasia. *N Engl J Med* 2000;
343:931–6.

Gardner-Medwin J, Dolezalova P,
Cummins C, Southwood TR.
Incidence of Henoch-Schönlein
purpura, Kawasaki disease, and
rare vasculitides in children of
different ethnic origins. *Lancet*
2002;360:1197–202.

Guttmacher AE, Marchuk DA,
White RI Jr. Hereditary hemorrhagic
telangiectasia. *N Engl J Med* 1995;
333:918–24.

Hood J, Burns CA, Hodges RE.
Sjogren's syndrome in scurvy. *N Engl
J Med* 1970;282:1120–4.

Peery WH. Clinical spectrum of
hereditary hemorrhagic telangiectasia
(Osler–Weber–Rendu Disease).
Am J Med 1987;82:989–97.

Pfeifer M, Boncristiano S, Bondolfi L
et al. Cerebral hemorrhage after
passive anti-A immunotherapy.
Science 2002;298:1379–80.

Press OW, Ramsey PG. Central nervous system infections associated with hereditary hemorrhagic telangiectasia. *Am J Med* 1984;77: 86–92.

Ronkainen J, Nuutinen M, Koskimies O. The adult kidney 24 years after childhood Henoch–Schönlein purpura: a retrospective cohort study. *Lancet* 2002;360:666–70.

Saba HI, Morelli GA, Logrono LA. Brief report: treatment of bleeding in hereditary hemorrhagic telangiectasia with aminocaproic acid. *N Engl J Med* 1994;330:1789–90.

Sabba C, Gallitelli M, Palasciano G. Efficacy of unusually high doses of tranexamic acid for the treatment of epistaxis in hereditary hemorrhagic telangiectasia. *N Engl J Med* 2001; 345:926.

Shetty AK, Steele RW, Silas V, Dehne R. A boy with a limp. *Lancet* 1998;351:182.

Swanson KL, Prakash BS, Stanson AW. Pulmonary arteriovenous fistulas: Mayo Clinic experience, 1982–1997. *Mayo Clin Proc* 1999;74:671–80.

Trembath RC, Thomson JR, Machado RD et al. Clinical and molecular genetic features of pulmonary hypertension in patients with hereditary hemorrhagic telangiectasia. *N Engl J Med* 2001;345:325–34.

Van Cutsem E, Piessevaux H. Pharmacologic therapy of arteriovenous malformations. *Gastrointest Endosc Clin N Am* 1996;6:819–32.

4 | Platelet disorders

Platelet function defects

Inherited disorders. Although uncommon, congenital platelet disorders have been described involving platelet membrane glycoproteins, storage granules and dense bodies. Some disorders (e.g. storage pool disorder) give rise to only relatively mild bleeding symptoms, and the diagnosis may not be made until the patient is well into adult life, usually following excessive bleeding after surgery (e.g. dental extraction) or trauma. Some of the congenital platelet disorders are also associated with morphologically abnormal platelets and thrombocytopenia.

Mutations in membrane glycoproteins. Bernard–Soulier syndrome is due to mutations in membrane Gp Ib-IX-V. The disorder is characterized by thrombocytopenia, large platelets and impaired binding of vWF. The last results in a prolonged bleeding time, defective platelet adhesion and poor platelet aggregation in response to ristocetin. The diagnosis should be suspected in patients with a history of bleeding and a reduced platelet count, and confirmed by reviewing the platelet morphology and observing abnormal ristocetin-induced aggregation, but normally functioning vWF. Desmopressin occasionally controls minor bleeding, but serious hemorrhage requires platelet infusions.

Glanzmann thrombasthenia is due to mutations in platelet membrane Gp IIb/IIIa, resulting in failure to bind fibrinogen. It is characterized by excessive menstrual blood loss, bleeding from mucous membranes, and major hemorrhage following trauma and surgery. The platelet count is normal, but clot retraction is greatly impaired and agents such as ADP, epinephrine and collagen fail to induce platelet aggregation. Platelet transfusions are usually needed to control bleeding. Women require hormonal therapy to control menorrhagia.

Defects in platelet storage organelles or granules. Platelet storage pool disease may be caused by the absence of dense bodies, which are the organelles containing ADP, ATP, calcium and serotonin. Excessive bruising and bleeding occurs after surgery or trauma as the platelets fail to exhibit a secondary wave of aggregation in response to a variety of aggregating agents. The absence of dense bodies in the platelets can be demonstrated by electron microscopy. Storage pool disease is often inherited together with tyrosinase-positive oculocutaneous albinism and ceroid pigment deposition in various organs, including the kidney. This constellation is termed the Hermansky–Pudlak syndrome and is due to mutations in *HPS1*, a gene coding for a vesicle coat-protein.

The gray platelet syndrome is characterized by a lack of platelet α-granules and absent platelet fibrinogen, fibronectin and thrombospondin. Some patients with this syndrome respond to treatment with desmopressin.

Cyclooxygenase defects result in impaired platelet aggregation in response to ADP, collagen and epinephrine, and may be associated with a mild bleeding tendency. Defects in platelet calcium mobilization are being more commonly recognized. Many other rare forms of inherited platelet dysfunction have been described, such as pseudo-vWD, collagen receptor deficiency, and the Chediak–Higashi and Wiskott–Aldrich syndromes.

Management. Patients with inherited platelet function defects should avoid aspirin and other drugs that alter platelet function. In addition, chronic blood loss may necessitate iron supplementation. Patients should carry documentation describing the nature of their bleeding defect with them at all times. If platelet transfusions are needed, single-donor platelets are usually preferred. If the patient becomes refractory to platelet transfusions, registries of Bernard–Soulier and Glanzmann patients indicate that recombinant human factor VIIa often provides satisfactory hemostasis, and the agent has received approval in the European Union for this indication.

Acquired disorders. Defective platelet function may be caused by alcohol, drugs, uremia and myeloproliferative disorders. Alcohol alone does not appear to affect platelet function, but strongly potentiates the inhibitory effects of aspirin. Antibiotics that inhibit bacterial cell wall synthesis, such as the penicillins and cephalosporins, appear to affect the platelet membrane and prolong the skin bleeding time. Minoxidil inhibits the synthesis of platelet prostaglandins. Valproic acid lowers the platelet count, prolongs the bleeding time and impairs platelet aggregation. The black tree fungus, used in Szechuan cooking, inhibits platelet aggregation. The effects of drugs used therapeutically (e.g. aspirin, clopidogrel) are discussed in Chapter 13 and uremic bleeding in Chapter 9.

Primary (essential) thrombocythemia is a myeloproliferative disorder that results from a clonal proliferation of stem cells. This proliferation primarily affects megakaryocyte production, resulting in an increase in the number of circulating platelets, which may have defective function. It is predominantly a disease of the elderly, but 20% of patients are less than 40 years of age, and more women than men are affected. Thrombotic events are more common than bleeding, which occurs in about 4% of patients. Bruises, bleeding gums and major gastrointestinal hemorrhage may occur. The spleen may be enlarged, and the peripheral blood smear often shows giant, agranular or hypogranular platelets. A variety of platelet function defects involving the platelet membrane, granules and enzymatic pathways have been described. Treatment in symptomatic patients is directed towards reducing the platelet count using agents such as hydroxyurea, radiophosphorus or α-interferon. Aspirin may reduce the risk of thrombotic events.

Thrombocytopenia

The normal platelet count ranges from 150×10^9/L to 350×10^9/L; thrombocytopenia is defined as a count of less than 150×10^9/L and may be mild, moderate or severe (Table 4.1). Bleeding seldom occurs with platelet counts greater than 50×10^9/L, and is usually minor with counts exceeding 10×10^9/L. Spontaneous bleeding and bleeding requiring medical attention usually indicate that the platelet count is less than 10×10^9/L. However, clinical bleeding often does not correlate with the platelet count because other factors, such as the integrity of the endothelium and the function of the residual platelets, also affect hemostasis.

Diagnosis. Careful scrutiny of a freshly prepared blood film is particularly helpful in the diagnosis of thrombocytopenia. The first step is to confirm that the platelet count is truly decreased and then

TABLE 4.1

Definition of thrombocytopenia

	Platelet count ($\times 10^9$/L)
Mild	50–150
Moderate	20–50
Severe	< 20

to detect whether other blood abnormalities are present. Pseudo-thrombocytopenia occurs when platelets undergo agglutination on exposure to cold, form satellites around leukocytes or clump in the presence of anticoagulants, such as ethylenediamine tetra-acetic acid (EDTA) or heparin. Under these conditions, automated counters do not recognize platelets and a spuriously low platelet count is recorded. However, clumps of platelets may be seen on the feather-edge of blood films indicating that the platelet count is higher than reported. In these circumstances, repeating the count using freshly drawn blood or using citrate anticoagulant may provide a more accurate estimate of platelet numbers. Examination of the blood smear will also provide information about platelet size. Large platelets are present in congenital thrombocytopenias, such as Bernard–Soulier syndrome and May–Hegglin anomaly (see Figure 2.2, page 20), or may indicate an increase in platelet turnover as in the immune thrombocytopenias and consumption syndromes. Small platelets occur in Wiskott–Aldrich syndrome. The red cells and white cells should also be examined: fragmented red cells may suggest a thrombotic microangiopathy, and hypogranular neutrophils suggest myelodysplasia.

Once a diagnosis of thrombocytopenia has been established, it is imperative to ascertain an exact etiology. Determining the time of onset of the condition by asking whether the patient ever had a normal platelet count helps to exclude congenital thrombocytopenias. A careful history to determine recent exposure to alcohol, herbal medications or other tonics, quinine water or unusual foods and other drugs may implicate a culprit agent. Viral infections, such as human immunodeficiency virus (HIV) or cytomegalovirus, are often associated with thrombocytopenia. Postoperative thrombocytopenias are usually dilutional, because replacement fluids lack platelets, and often resolve within a few days. On the other hand, thrombocytopenias associated with cardiac surgery, the use of aortic balloon pump devices or leaky heart valves may be persistent, and may not improve until the pump is removed or the valve repaired. Severe thrombocytopenia may result from the use of platelet glycoprotein inhibitors during coronary angioplasty and stenting. If such features are absent from the history, an immune thrombocytopenia is most likely. Most often this an autoimmune disorder, such as immune thrombocytopenic purpura (ITP), but other possibilities such as antiphospholipid antibody syndrome and post-transfusion purpura should be considered.

In evaluating a patient with thrombocytopenia, it is useful to consider the clinical setting (Table 4.2). For example, a young woman presenting with new onset of bleeding from the nose and mouth, vaginal bleeding and petechiae probably has ITP, whereas an asymptomatic pregnant woman with a platelet count of 100×10^9/L probably has benign incidental thrombocytopenia. An acute decline in platelet count in a patient undergoing treatment for cardiac, rheumatological or infectious disease suggests that a drug may be responsible (see page 43). Thrombocytopenia in association with an acute illness, such as sepsis or acute respiratory distress syndrome, usually indicates platelet consumption, and may be accompanied by signs of DIC. Thrombocytopenia accompanied by microangiopathic hemolytic anemia and evidence of thrombosis warrants a consideration of thrombotic thrombocytopenic purpura (TTP), hemolytic–uremic syndrome (HUS), or heparin-induced thrombocytopenia (HIT). On the other hand, a previously healthy person who presents with pancytopenia may have aplastic anemia or leukemia; enlargement of the spleen might suggest liver disease, myelofibrosis or a storage disorder, such as Gaucher disease.

Immune thrombocytopenic purpura was previously thought to affect mostly young women but, with the aging of the population, it is increasingly being recognized in the elderly, with men and women

TABLE 4.2

Differential diagnosis of thrombocytopenia

Cause of thrombocytopenia	Setting	Observations
Immune (autoantibodies)	Young woman	Appears healthy
Drug-induced	Other illness	Drugs (e.g. gold, quinidine; see page 44)
Acute respiratory distress syndrome	Intensive care unit	Normal PT, APTT, fibrinogen
Disseminated intravascular coagulation	Sepsis, malignancy	Abnormal PT, APTT, fibrinogen
Thrombotic microangiopathy/ thrombotic thrombocytopenic purpura	Seizure, renal disease	Fragmented red cells
HELLP syndrome	Pregnancy	Abnormal liver enzymes
Heparin-induced thrombocytopenia	Thrombosis	Heparin
Aplastic anemia	Bleeding, infection	Anemia, neutropenia
Liver disease, myeloproliferative	Chronic disease	Splenomegaly

APTT, activated partial thromboplastin time; HELLP, hemolytic anemia with elevated liver enzymes and low platelet count; PT, prothrombin time.

equally affected. The overall incidence is 2.5/100 000 but, in those over 60, it increases to 4.5/100 000.

Diagnosis. In many patients, the thrombocytopenia is discovered when a complete blood count is performed as part of a periodic health examination; however, others may notice a petechial rash or oral bleeding and consult their physician. A complete history should be obtained, focusing on whether symptoms such as fever, pain or weight loss are present, recent respiratory infections or HIV risk factors, and

consumption of alcohol or tonic water containing quinine. Detailed
inquiry should be made about recent exposure to drugs or herbal
medicines. On physical examination, signs of bleeding such as petechiae
(Figure 4.1), subconjunctival hemorrhage (Figure 4.2), ecchymoses and
hemorrhagic bullae in the oral cavity should be sought. Evidence of
systemic disorders, such as signs of recent weight loss, hypothyroidism,
lymphadenopathy and splenomegaly, should also be noted. A complete
blood count indicates the severity of the thrombocytopenia; a
concomitant hypochromic, microcytic anemia may be present if
bleeding has been chronic, but the leukocyte count is generally normal.

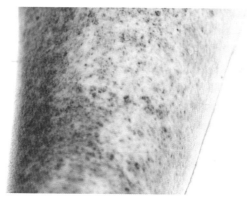

Figure 4.1 Petechiae in immune thrombocytopenic purpura.

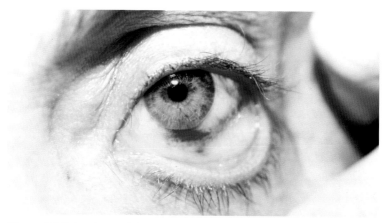

Figure 4.2 Subconjunctival hemorrhage in a patient with immune
thrombocytopenic purpura.

As noted previously, examination of the blood film is mandatory to confirm the thrombocytopenia and exclude other hematologic disorders. If the history, physical examination or blood count are normal, no further evaluations are necessary according to the *Guidelines for the Management of ITP* published by the American Society of Hematology. However, a bone marrow examination is recommended in those over 60 years of age, as it may be difficult to distinguish ITP from myelodysplasia in the elderly. Also, tests for occult thyroid disease or HIV may be appropriate in some situations.

Treatment. If the platelet count is greater than $50 \times 10^9/L$, no treatment is required and patients may simply be observed at regular intervals. In children, ITP is usually an acute, self-limiting condition and, provided there is no frank or persistent bleeding, drug therapy may not be necessary. In adults, however, the thrombocytopenia may be more prolonged and specific treatment may be required. Table 4.3 shows some of the agents used for the management of symptomatic ITP. If the platelet count is less than $30 \times 10^9/L$ or there is bleeding,

TABLE 4.3

Treatment of acute immune thrombocytopenic purpura

Agent	Dose	Comment
Prednisone	1 mg/kg/day	Response time 5–7 days
Methylprednisolone	Day 1, 30 mg/kg i.v.; day 2, 15 mg/kg i.v.	Infuse over 30 minutes; monitor for seizures, hypokalemia
Anti-D immunoglobulin	50–75 µg/kg i.v.	Causes hemolysis; ineffective in rhesus negative patients and after splenectomy
Immunoglobulin G	1 g/kg/day i.v. for 2 days	Infuse over 4–6 hours to avoid allergic reactions; monitor renal function
Rituximab	375 mg/m^2/week i.v. for 4 weeks	Adverse reactions include fever, chills, infections

prednisone, 1 mg/kg, should be given. Patients with platelet counts of less than 20×10^9/L are generally hospitalized; if there is considerable bleeding, methylprednisolone may be given intravenously. Because the response to oral steroids may take 5–7 days, many physicians prescribe immunoglobulin in addition to corticosteroids. In children, if treatment is indicated, intravenous IgG is often used in the USA, whereas treatment with steroids is usually initiated in the UK.

If the patient is rhesus positive, has a hemoglobin level above 100 g/L and has not previously had a splenectomy, anti-D immunoglobulin, 50–75 µg/kg intravenously, may be given. Alternatively, patients may be given intravenous IgG, 1 g/kg/day for 2 days or 400 mg/kg/day for 5 days; intravenous IgG should always be given slowly, over 4–6 hours, to avoid anaphylactic reactions. Renal function should also be monitored as renal failure induced by intravenous IgG has been reported; this is a result of the high sucrose content of early preparations, and a lower incidence has been reported for more recent preparations manufactured without the addition of sucrose. Responses to anti-D immunoglobulin or intravenous IgG usually occur within 24–48 hours, but relapses are common in adult patients.

Once the platelet count has increased to over 30×10^9/L, the dose of corticosteroid is tapered slowly to avoid a rapid relapse. The goal is to prevent recurrence of bleeding by maintaining the platelet count above 20×10^9/L. If the dose of corticosteroid required to accomplish this is greater than 10–20 mg/day, other interventions, such as pulsed dexamethasone, rituximab or splenectomy, may be required. Every effort should be made to delay splenectomy as long as possible, since this is an irreversible step that places the patient at lifelong risk of fatal sepsis. As early as possible before surgery, patients are immunized against pneumococcal infection and *Haemophilus influenzae* and, in some centers, meningococcal vaccines are given. Preoperatively, the platelet count is raised by administering high doses of corticosteroid. Methylprednisolone, up to 30 mg/kg, may be given by slow intravenous infusion daily for 1–2 days; the platelet count will often increase to more than 50×10^9/L within 48 hours. Other treatments for refractory ITP include rituximab, danazol, vincristine, cyclophosphamide and ciclosporin (Table 4.4).

TABLE 4.4

Treatment of chronic immune thrombocytopenic purpura

Agent	Dose	Adverse effects
Dexamethasone	40 mg/day orally for 4 days, every 28 days	Excitability, hyperglycemia, hypokalemia
Rituximab	375 mg/m^2/week i.v. for 4 weeks	Fever, chills, infections
Danazol	200 mg four times daily orally	Amenorrhea, hirsutism, cholestatic hepatitis
Vincristine	1–2 mg/week i.v.	Phlebitis, skin necrosis, neuropathy, SIADH
Cyclophosphamide	1–1.5 g/m^2 i.v. every 4 weeks	Leukopenia, cystitis
Ciclosporin	2.5–3 mg/kg/day	Renal failure, hypertension

SIADH, syndrome of inappropriate release of antidiuretic hormone.

Thrombotic microangiopathies are not bleeding disorders, but are accompanied by thrombocytopenia and include TTP, HUS, *h*emolytic anemia with *e*levated *l*iver enzymes and *l*ow *p*latelet count (HELLP) syndrome in pregnancy, and HIT. The clinical picture reflects ischemic injury to one or more organs or tissues: the brain, heart and kidney in TTP; the kidney in HUS; the liver in HELLP; and limb or bowel gangrene in HIT. Laboratory evaluation reveals microangiopathic hemolytic anemia with red cell fragmentation and reticulocytosis, thrombocytopenia and raised levels of lactic dehydrogenase (LDH). TTP is treated by plasma exchange, HUS by withdrawal of drugs (ciclosporin) or removal of Shiga toxins, HELLP by delivery of the fetus and placenta, and HIT by cessation of heparin and administration of antithrombotic agents, such as direct thrombin inhibitors.

Thrombocytopenia in pregnancy (see Chapter 10). Thrombocytopenia is observed in 7–8% of pregnancies. It is usually a benign, incidental finding, but may be associated with hypertensive disorders of pregnancy, a manifestation of ITP or a pseudo-thrombocytopenia due to platelet clumping in vitro. Pseudo-thrombocytopenia can be excluded by examining the peripheral smear for platelet clumps. The true platelet count can be assessed by platelet quantitation immediately after the blood is drawn, as the platelets may agglutinate while the blood is standing at room temperature. Occasionally, drawing the blood into citrate anticoagulant, rather than EDTA, will provide a more accurate platelet count.

Once it has been established that the patient has a true thrombocytopenia, the benign, gestational thrombocytopenias that account for 70% of cases must be differentiated from the uncommon ITP that accounts for 4% of cases (Table 4.5).

Benign gestational thrombocytopenia does not require treatment; observation alone is adequate. However, ITP during pregnancy may be severe. Monthly infusions of intravenous IgG may be needed to

TABLE 4.5

Differential diagnosis of thrombocytopenia in pregnancy*

Observation	Gestational thrombocytopenia	Immune thrombocytopenic purpura
History of thrombocytopenia	Only during pregnancy	Present between pregnancies
Platelet count	Generally > 70×10^9/L; stable during pregnancy	Usually < 70×10^9/L; progressively declines during pregnancy
Tests of autoimmunity (e.g. ANA, ACA)	Negative	Often positive
Neonatal thrombocytopenia	No	Up to 10% of fetuses have thrombocytopenia (platelets < 50×10^9/L)

*See also Chapter 10.
ACA, anticardiolipin antibody; ANA, antinuclear antibody.

prevent bleeding. A platelet count should be obtained from the infant, preferably from the cord blood, immediately after delivery, and repeated daily for the first week. If the infant has a platelet count of less than 20×10^9/L or is bleeding, intravenous IgG infusions are given. The thrombocytopenia usually resolves within 1–2 weeks. Neonatal alloimmune thrombocytopenia is discussed in Chapter 10 (page 88).

Thrombocytopenia associated with HIV. Thrombocytopenia is a common complication in patients with HIV infection, but spontaneous bleeding is rare, even if the platelet count is severely depressed. Several mechanisms for the thrombocytopenia have been established, including platelet antibodies and viral infection of megakaryocytes. In the later stages of infection, atrophy of the marrow may occur, with pancytopenia. Platelet counts will often increase gradually with institution of effective anti-retroviral therapy. A more rapid increase in platelet count occurs with infusions of anti-D or intravenous IgG.

Iatrogenic causes of thrombocytopenia

Drug-induced thrombocytopenia is uncommon; an annual incidence of 18 cases/million population has been reported. In 1998, George et al. conducted a systematic review of published cases of drug-induced thrombocytopenia, and provided an update in February 2001. A total of 104 drugs were found to have a definite or probable causal role. Quinidine was listed in 38 reports, gold in 11 and co-trimoxazole in 10. Major bleeding was documented in 9% of cases and death in 0.8%. Drugs for which there was strong evidence of involvement are listed in Table 4.6.

Many other agents, including pulped sesame seeds and Chinese herbal medicines, may cause acute thrombocytopenia. TTP has been induced by ticlopidine, presumably by stimulating antibodies against ADAMST-13, the protease that inactivates vWF.

Non-drug causes of thrombocytopenia include exposure to thrombopoietin and post-transfusion purpura. When volunteers were given a preparation of recombinant thrombopoietin, they developed antibodies that prevented native thrombopoietin from binding to

TABLE 4.6

Examples of drugs that cause thrombocytopenia and bleeding

- Amiodarone
- Atorvastatin
- Carbamazepine
- Chlorpropamide
- Cimetidine
- Diclofenac
- Digoxin
- Glycoprotein IIb/IIIa inhibitors
  (e.g. abciximab, tirofiban)
- Gold
- Indinavir

- Mesaline
- Methyldopa
- Nalidixic acid
- Quinidine and quinine
- Pentoxifylline
- Procainamide
- Ranitidine
- Rifampin
- Co-trimoxazole
- Vancomycin

its receptor, impairing platelet production and inducing severe thrombocytopenia. Post-transfusion purpura occurs when individuals lacking the platelet PL^{AI} antigen, an antigen present in over 97% of the population, are transfused with blood products containing this antigen. A strong antibody response occurs and the antibodies cross-react with the patient's own platelets, producing a severe thrombocytopenia. Thrombocytopenia has even occurred when organs from a PL^{AI} antigen-negative individual are transplanted into a PL^{AI} antigen-positive recipient; the antibody response is presumably mediated by donor lymphocytes carried within the organs.

Pathogenesis of drug-induced thrombocytopenia. A variety of mechanisms underlie drug-induced thrombocytopenia, including binding to the platelet membrane glycoproteins and stimulating the production of hapten-dependent antibodies that recognize drug–protein targets. Heparin induces a conformational change in platelet factor 4, exposing neoantigens, which elicit antibodies. Other drugs, such as quinidine and sulfonamides, induce antibodies that bind to platelet glycoproteins in the presence of the drug or one of its metabolites. Some bind to the glycoproteins in the absence of the drug.

Abciximab, a 'humanized' mouse monoclonal antibody directed against Gp IIb/IIIa, may stimulate antibodies that react with abciximab-coated platelets and are specific for murine protein. Finally, small molecule inhibitors of platelet Gp IIb/IIIa elicit antibodies that recognize multiple epitopes on the glycoprotein when it is complexed with the inhibitor; these antibodies may be directed against the ligand binding site.

Management. All new medications or tonics should be discontinued, and serial platelet counts obtained. If the patient is not bleeding, watchful waiting is appropriate. However, major or life-threatening hemorrhage necessitates platelet infusion. Important exceptions are thrombocytopenia associated with heparin and TTP; in these disorders, infused platelets worsen the thromboses and are contraindicated.

Platelet transfusions are indicated to:

- control bleeding due to decreased platelet numbers or impaired platelet function
- correct dilutional thrombocytopenia resulting from multi-unit transfusion of packed red cells in conjunction with surgery or trauma
- prevent bleeding in individuals with thrombocytopenia and recent bleeding into vital structures
- prevent bleeding in thrombocytopenic persons undergoing invasive procedures
- prevent bleeding in patients with platelet counts of less than 10×10^9/L and impaired platelet production due to:
  - marrow replacement by malignancies
  - marrow depletion by chemotherapy or radiation
  - marrow impairment associated with hematopoietic cell transplantation.

Platelets may be obtained by plateletpheresis (single-donor platelets) or retrieved from donated whole blood (random-donor platelets). One apheresis unit is equivalent to six random-donor units in terms of platelet numbers. Each random-donor unit generally increases the platelet count by 5×10^9/L, so that one apheresis unit or six random-donor units should provide a satisfactory increase in platelet count, but this must be verified by performing a platelet count 1 hour and 24 hours after the infusion. This will also give some indication of the recovery and survival of the infused platelets. Infusion of platelets can be associated with allergic reactions, which can be minimized by depleting the platelets of accompanying white cells. Transmission of infectious agents may also occur; careful donor screening may reduce some of this risk. Platelet products must also be screened for bacterial contamination. Platelet sensitization is uncommon, even with random-donor platelets; if platelet alloimmunization develops, platelet cross-matching and giving human leukocyte antigen (HLA)-matched platelets may be helpful.

Key points – platelet disorders

- Thrombocytopenia may occur with some inherited disorders of platelet function, such as the Bernard–Soulier, gray platelet and Wiskott–Aldrich syndromes.
- Inhibitors of platelet function, such as aspirin, should be avoided in individuals with disorders of platelet function and those with thrombocytopenia.
- In immune thrombocytopenia, bleeding is uncommon if the platelet count exceeds 10×10^9/L and aggressive interventions (e.g. high-dose corticosteroids, splenectomy) are not usually indicated.
- The drugs most commonly implicated in immune thrombo-cytopenia are quinidine, co-trimoxazole and gold.
- Platelet transfusion has limited indications and should be used sparingly, because it may transmit infection or sensitize the recipient to platelet antigens.

Key references

Allford SL, Hunt BJ, Rose P et al. Guidelines on the diagnosis and management of the thrombotic microangiopathic haemolytic anaemias. *Br J Haematol* 2003;120:556–73.

Aster RH. Drug-induced immune thrombocytopenia: an overview of pathogensis. *Semin Hematol* 1999;36(suppl 1):2–6. (See also: *Blood* 2002;99:2054–9 and *Blood* 2002;100:2071–6.)

British Committee for Standards in Haematology General Haematology Task Force. Guidelines for the investigation and management of idiopathic thrombocytopenic purpura in adults, children and in pregnancy. *Br J Haematol* 2003; 120:574–96.

George JN. Platelets. *Lancet* 2000;355:1531–9.

George JN, Raskob GE, Shah SR et al. Drug-induced thrombocytopenia: a systematic review of published case reports. *Ann Intern Med* 1998;129:886–90. (Update: *Ann Intern Med* 2001;134:346.)

George JN, Woolf SH, Raskob GE et al. Idiopathic thrombocytopenic purpura: a practice guideline developed by explicit methods for the American Society of Hematology. *Blood* 1996;88:3–40.

Gill KK, Kelton JG. Management of ITP in pregnancy. *Semin Hematol* 2000;37:275–89.

Kaufman DW, Kelly JP, Johannes CB et al. Acute thrombocytopenic purpura in relation to the use of drugs. *Blood* 1993;82:2714–18.

McMillan R. Therapy for adults with refractory chronic immune thrombocytopenic purpura. *Ann Intern Med* 1997;126:307–14.

Olkkonen VM, Ikonen E. Genetic defects of intracellular-membrane transport. *N Engl J Med* 2000;343: 1095–104.

Scaradavou A, Woo B, Woloski BM et al. Intravenous anti-D treatment of immune thrombocytopenic purpura: experience in 272 patients. *Blood* 1997;89:2689–700.

Schiffer CA, Anderson KC, Bennett CL et al. Platelet transfusion for patients with cancer: clinical practice guidelines of the American Society of Clinical Oncology. *J Clin Oncol* 2001;19:1519–38.

Shrimpton CN, Andrews RK, Lopez JA, Berndt MC. Congenital disorders of platelet function. In: Loscalzo J, Schafer AI, eds. *Thrombosis and Hemorrhage*. 3rd edn. Philadelphia: Lippincott Williams & Wilkins, 2002: 507–24.

Tefferi A, ed. Recent advances in the treatment of essential thrombocythemia. *Semin Hematol* 1999;36(suppl 2):1–29.

In a bleeding state due to a clotting factor deficiency, the aim of treatment is to raise the level of the deficient factor. However, there are some drugs that have a more non-specific effect in promoting hemostasis by preventing the lysis of the developing platelet/fibrin plug by the fibrinolytic system or stimulating the release of clotting factors.

This chapter considers the use of fibrinolytic inhibitors, which have a well-defined place in the management of a variety of different bleeding conditions, and the vasopressin analog, desmopressin, which raises factor VIII and vWF levels. Although desmopressin is used primarily to treat hemophilia A and vWD, it is also effective in a number of other situations.

Tranexamic acid and ε-aminocaproic acid

Tranexamic acid and EACA are synthetic amino acids that inhibit fibrinolysis by binding to the lysine-binding site on plasminogen and preventing it from interacting with its substrate, fibrin (Figure 5.1). They should be used with caution in those at high risk of myocardial infarction, stroke or DIC.

Primary menorrhagia. In the absence of an organic lesion in the uterus, tranexamic acid may have a role in reducing menstrual loss because fibrinolytic activity is strongly expressed by the endometrium. It is usual to attempt control of menorrhagia initially with estrogen–progestogen preparations but, if these fail or are contraindicated, tranexamic acid may be effective.

Gastrointestinal bleeding. The stomach has a high concentration of fibrinolytic enzymes and there is evidence that tranexamic acid reduces upper gastrointestinal bleeding. It is usually only used as an adjuvant to another more specific therapy (e.g. endoscopic injection of adrenaline [epinephrine] into the base of a bleeding peptic ulcer).

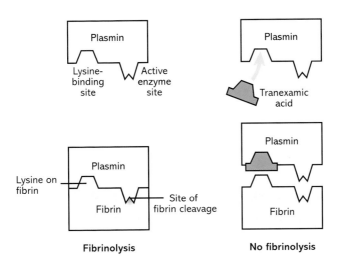

Figure 5.1 Mechanism of inhibition of fibrinolysis by tranexamic acid. The plasmin binding site on fibrin contains a lysine residue. In the absence of tranexamic acid, the plasmin binds, resulting in cleavage of fibrin. Tranexamic acid, an analog of lysine, binds to plasmin and sterically prevents it from binding to fibrin and thus prevents fibrinolysis.

Bleeding in the urinary tract. Dissolution of clots in the urinary tract is promoted by urokinase secreted by the kidney. This fibrinolytic activity in urine, however, tends to exacerbate any tendency to bleed, such as after prostatectomy or if a bladder polyp is present. In these circumstances, tranexamic acid inhibits urokinase and can reduce bleeding from the bladder. It should, however, never be given if there is a possibility of bleeding into the ureter or kidney because, if a clot forms in the ureter, it may not be lysed and may cause obstructive uropathy.

Bleeding disorders. In most patients with congenital (e.g. hemophilia) or acquired bleeding disorders, the appropriate way to manage bleeding or potential bleeding (e.g. after surgery) is to raise the plasma level of the deficient clotting factor. However, the addition of a fibrinolytic inhibitor can help maintain hemostasis. Tranexamic acid has a well-defined role after dental extraction; it should be given orally in a dose of 15 mg/kg every 8 hours for 10 days and can also be used as a mouthwash (50 mg/mL) in the immediate postoperative period.

Tranexamic acid or EACA may also be used to prevent postoperative bleeding in patients with thrombocytopenia who require minor surgery.

Aprotinin

Aprotinin is a small polypeptide extracted from beef lung that inhibits serine proteases; kallikrein, which activates factor XII and thus both coagulation and fibrinolysis, can be inhibited by aprotinin. It has an accepted place during cardiac surgery, particularly for patients taking aspirin or with other preexisting hemostatic defects, patients with endocarditis, patients requiring reoperation and patients undergoing heart transplantation. It also has a place in reducing the use of blood during orthotopic liver transplantation.

Desmopressin

Desmopressin (1-deamino-8-D-arginine vasopressin) is a vasopressin analog that increases the plasma levels of factor VIII and vWF 3–5-fold. The ability to raise the level of factor VIII and vWF makes desmopressin particularly useful for treating patients with mild hemophilia A and vWD, especially when short-term therapy is required (Figure 5.2). For example, to cover dental surgery, it is only necessary to raise the level of the deficient factor to about 50% normal for 4–6 hours, and lysis of the formed clots can be prevented with a fibrinolytic inhibitor. Desmopressin is usually given intravenously in a dose of 0.3 µg/kg over 15 minutes. Peak factor VIII and vWF levels are observed after 30–60 minutes. Further doses can be given after 4–6 hours, but the response is usually diminished (tachyphylaxis). Desmopressin also has a place in the treatment of other congenital bleeding disorders (e.g. platelet storage pool disorder) and some acquired conditions (e.g. renal failure). Water retention, and consequent hyponatremia, may complicate desmopressin therapy, particularly in children. It is prudent to monitor the serum sodium if it is anticipated that more than one dose of the drug will be needed.

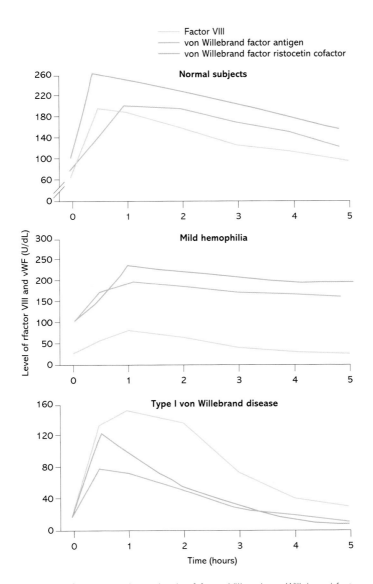

Figure 5.2 Changes in plasma levels of factor VIII and von Willebrand factor (vWF) after an intravenous infusion of desmopressin in normal subjects, patients with mild hemophilia and patients with type 1 von Willebrand's disease. A post-infusion level of 50 IU/dL is adequate to treat bleeds or cover surgery. Reproduced with permission from Ludlam CA et al. *Br J Haematol* 1980; 45:499–511.

Key points – hemostatic products

- Tranexamic acid and ε-aminocaproic acid (EACA) are useful for preventing hemorrhage following dental and other surgery, and to treat menorrhagia.
- Tranexamic acid or EACA should not be given to patients with disseminated intravascular coagulation or those who may be bleeding from the upper urinary tract.
- Desmopressin is often effective hemostatic therapy in mild hemophilia A, von Willebrand's disease and some platelet disorders.
- The antidiuretic effect of desmopressin lasts for 24 hours and can lead to clinically significant water retention and hyponatremia.

Key references

Green D, Sanders J, Eiken M et al. Recombinant aprotinin in coronary artery bypass graft surgery. *J Thorac Cardiovasc Surg* 1995;110:963–70.

Kaufmann JE, Vischer UM. Cellular mechanisms of the hemostatic effects of desmopressin (DDAVP). *J Thromb Haemost* 2003;1:682–9.

Mannucci PM. Desmopressin in the treatment of bleeding disorders: the first twenty years. *Blood* 1997; 90:2515–21.

Mannucci PM. Haemostatic drugs. *N Engl J Med* 1998;339:245–53.

Hemophilia A and B are the most common severe congenital bleeding disorders and result from a deficiency of coagulation factors VIII and IX, respectively. The genes for both these conditions are located on the X chromosome; they are, therefore, sex-linked disorders that almost exclusively affect males. Female carriers may, however, have reduced plasma levels of factors VIII and IX, and therefore have a mild bleeding disorder. Hemophilia A is about five times more common than hemophilia B. Clinically, the conditions have an identical presentation and can only be distinguished by measuring plasma levels of the specific clotting factors. The bleeding potential, or clinical severity, is directly related to plasma levels of factors VIII and IX (Table 6.1); those with levels below 1 IU/dL (< 1% of normal) have severe hemophilia and the most frequent bleeds.

Molecular genetics of hemophilia A and B. The causative mutations for hemophilia A and B are found in the genes for factors VIII and IX, respectively. The factor VIII gene is large at 186 kb in length and this accounts for its greater risk of mutation (and therefore higher prevalence of hemophilia A) compared with that of factor IX, which is only 34 kb. A large number of different mutations have been described associated with varying reductions in factor VIII/IX activity. Major

TABLE 6.1

Clinical severity of hemophilia A and B

Severity	Level of factors VIII and IX (IU/dL)	Clinical presentation
Mild	> 5	Postoperative or severe post-traumatic bleeds
Moderate	2–5	Bleeds after mild trauma
Severe	< 1	'Spontaneous' bleeds

disruption of either gene leads to severe hemophilia, whereas minor defects, such as a single base change, often result in a molecule that retains some of its functional activity and causes only mild hemophilia. About 50% of cases of severe hemophilia A result from a major inversion in intron 22 of the gene with a homologous region of the chromosome at 400 kb distant (known as the 'flip-tip' inversion, Figure 6.1). In those without a family history, this inversion may have occurred in meiosis during spermatogenesis in the patient's grandfather. In the laboratory, with the current polymerase chain reaction and gene

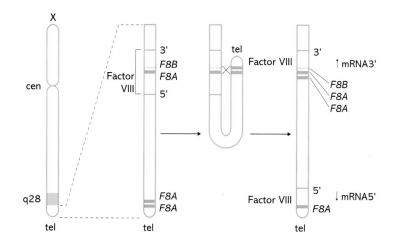

Figure 6.1 The 'flip-tip' rearrangement of the factor VIII gene is responsible for up to 50% of cases of severe hemophilia A. On the X chromosome, there are three copies of a gene *F8A*, which is of unknown function. One copy is within intron 22 of the factor VIII gene, and two copies are in the opposite orientation and situated 400 kb telomeric to the factor VIII gene. During meiosis in spermatogenesis, the long arm of the X chromosome does not have a homologous chromosome to pair with and, instead, there is occasionally an intrachromosomal pairing with a subsequent crossover. Crossovers can occur with either the proximal or distal distant F8A gene, leading to two separately transcribed mRNAs, neither of which codes for functional factor VIII. Reprinted with permission from Elsevier (Tuddenham EG. *Lancet*, 1994;343:308).

sequencing techniques, it is now possible to characterize the mutation in each family. It is important to do this, because the clinical features are related to the mutation (e.g. the likelihood of antifactor VIII antibody developing following treatment is higher with certain mutations), and because it makes identification of female carriers in the family much more straightforward.

Clinical features

If the mother is a known carrier or there is a family history of hemophilia, boys can be tested at birth by measuring the plasma levels of factors VIII and IX. For other patients, the age at presentation will depend on the severity of the hemophilia.

Those with severe hemophilia usually experience their first bleed at about 6–9 months of age, when they start to become mobile and develop hemarthroses. Some present earlier, particularly if they receive an intramuscular injection and a muscle hematoma develops, or they experience other surgery or trauma, for example, to the frenulum of the tongue. Many bleeds in patients with severe hemophilia are apparently spontaneous, without a history of trauma, and may occur once or twice weekly.

Boys with mild or moderate hemophilia usually present later, the age depending on the levels of factors VIII and IX. Those with mild hemophilia may not be diagnosed until young adult life when they are likely to be exposed to greater trauma. When circumcision, tonsillectomy and dental extractions were common procedures in childhood, mild and moderate hemophilia were often diagnosed as a result of postoperative bleeding. Those with moderate hemophilia bleed after minor trauma more often (about once a month), while those with mild hemophilia only bleed after major trauma or surgery.

Sites of bleeding

Joints. The most common sites for bleeds are the knees, elbows, ankles, hips and shoulders. Hemorrhage occurs from the synovium into the joint cavity, though it may spread outside, particularly if the capsule has been injured by trauma. The patient is usually aware that a bleed is starting before there are any signs of swelling or limitation of movement. Untreated bleeding continues until the joint is tense, swollen and exceedingly painful. The blood within the joint space causes a strong inflammatory reaction: there is marked vasodilatation and leukocyte enzymes erode the cartilage; and the synovium hypertrophies and becomes friable. These pathophysiological changes predispose to further hemorrhage. Muscle atrophy around the joint leads to instability and further predisposes to bleeding. Unless treated early and adequately, several bleeds into a joint will weaken it considerably (Figure 6.2). When this happens, it is known as a 'target joint'. Eventually, the cartilage becomes completely eroded and secondary osteoarthritis develops.

Without adequate and prompt treatment, patients with severe hemophilia develop progressive degenerative arthrosis of the knees, elbow, hips and ankles, and eventually become severely physically disabled. Regular prophylactic therapy two or three times weekly in childhood, however, prevents hemarthroses and enables children to grow up with near normal joints.

Muscles. Muscle hematomas are also characteristic of hemophilia. The large weight-bearing muscles are most commonly affected, particularly the iliopsoas, calf, gluteal and forearm muscles. Bleeding is often insidious and may have been occurring for some time before discomfort is noticed; as a result, patients eventually present with a large hematoma. If the muscle is surrounded by an inflexible fascial sheath and bleeding continues unchecked, the resultant increase in pressure causes a compartment syndrome with impairment of the blood supply, tissue ischemia, necrosis, and subsequent fibrosis and muscle shortening. When this occurs in the calf, the shortening of the muscle pulls up the Achilles tendon, making it impossible for the patient to put his heel on the ground. As a consequence, he has to walk on the ball of the foot and this leads to forefoot deformity.

Bleeding into the iliopsoas muscle characteristically presents with pain in the groin or iliac fossa, flexion of the hip joint and parasthesia in the anterior thigh over the distribution of the femoral nerve. This triad of symptoms arises because the muscle becomes swollen as it passes under the anterior ligament and presses on the femoral nerve; flexion reduces pressure in the muscle and on the nerve.

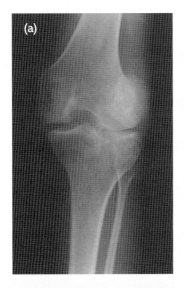

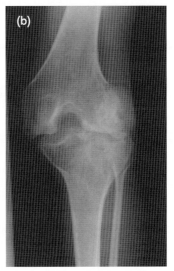

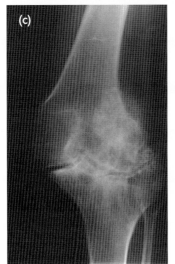

Figure 6.2 Radiograph of the knee of patient with severe hemophilia. (a) As a young adult demonstrating deformity, loss of joint space over the lateral tibial plate and sclerosis of the bone. (b) Further loss of cartilage and squaring up on the intercondylar notch. (c) Total loss of cartilage, marked sclerosis and bony cysts.

Brain. Intracranial bleeds are an uncommon, but serious, complication. They may be precipitated by mild trauma, but can occur apparently spontaneously. Bleeding is usually into the substance of the cerebrum. Patients present with dizziness, vomiting, headache and loss of consciousness, and examination reveals clinical evidence of raised intracranial pressure.

Surgery. In an undiagnosed hemophiliac, bleeding may not be excessive at operation, but persistent oozing leads to a large hematoma after 3–4 days. After dental extractions, bleeding may be delayed for 4–6 hours, but then usually resumes and persists for days to weeks.

Treatment

Once bleeding has started, it is important to raise the level of factor VIII or IX promptly to arrest hemorrhage (Table 6.2). Treatment should be continued until bleeding has stopped. Further treatment may be necessary to prevent rebleeding during mobilization and physiotherapy.

In some patients with mild hemophilia, desmopressin, 0.3 µg/kg, may be capable of increasing factor VIII to the necessary level and it avoids the use of a clotting factor concentrate. In all other circumstances, a concentrate of either factor VIII or IX should be given. These concentrates are prepared from pooled donor plasma or by

TABLE 6.2

Plasma levels of factors VIII and IX that need to be achieved with therapy to treat bleeds*

	Hemophilia A		Hemophilia B	
	Plasma factor VIII (IU/dL)	Dose (IU/kg)	Plasma factor IX (IU/dL)	Dose (IU/kg)
Early, mild hemarthrosis	15–20	10–15	15–20	20–30
Severe hemarthrosis, especially after trauma	30–50	15–25	30–50	30–50
Surgery, major trauma, intracranial bleed	80–120	40–60	50–70	50–70

*Following infusion of factor IX, a proportion binds to endothelial cells resulting in a reduced in-vivo recovery compared with factor VIII. Thus, to achieve comparable levels, higher doses of factor IX are required.

recombinant technology. Plasma-derived concentrates contain predominantly either factor VIII (some also contain vWF) or IX, though they also contain small amounts of other plasma proteins, including albumin. Some recombinant factor VIII concentrates may also contain human and animal proteins that are used in the cell culture medium during manufacture, during purification or as an excipient in the final preparation. Recombinant factor VIII and IX concentrates are now available that are manufactured entirely without the addition of any human or animal protein.

Inhibitors

About a third of patients with severe hemophilia A develop an inhibitory IgG antibody against factor VIII concentrate after treatment. On average, this arises after about ten exposures to the concentrate. Many of the antibodies are transient, are present at low levels and spontaneously disappear after a short period, while others are present at higher levels and may persist. Treatment can be problematic in those patients with higher levels of antibody, because the infused factor VIII is immediately neutralized and therapy is ineffective. In such cases, recombinant human factor VIIa or activated prothrombin concentrate can be given. Both these concentrates are 'activated' and have hemostatic activity in patients with inhibitors. These treatments are not, however, as effective as factor VIII in a patient without an inhibitor. In many patients who develop inhibitors, it is possible to induce tolerance to factor VIII by giving regular daily infusions, even in the absence of bleeding, and the antibody becomes undetectable after 6–12 months. While inhibitors are rare in those with hemophilia B, tolerance is often much more difficult to establish.

Female carriers

Female carriers of hemophilia A and B may be identifiable from the family history alone. For example, a daughter of a hemophiliac, or a woman who has either two sons with hemophilia or one son and another hemophiliac in her extended family, are obligate carriers of hemophilia. Other women in families with a hemophiliac may be carriers; carrier status can be ascertained by assessment for the presence or absence of the mutation that is present in an affected family member. Alternatively, intragenic factor VIII/IX polymorphisms can be used to track the hemophilia gene in the family. Provided the X chromosome that carries the hemophilia gene can be distinguished from the X chromosome carrying the normal factor VIII gene (by the use of an intragenic polymorphism or known causative mutation in the family), antenatal diagnosis can be undertaken at about 11 weeks' gestation by chorionic villus sampling.

Infections transmitted by clotting factor concentrates

Clotting factor concentrates, currently prepared from donors screened for HIV, and hepatitis B and C, are virally attenuated by either heat or a solvent/detergent step in their manufacture, and no longer transmit these viruses. However, some infectious agents, such as parvovirus and prions, may resist inactivation and may have the potential to be transmitted by transfusion. Routine vaccination against hepatitis A and B when hemophilia is diagnosed also helps to prevent infection.

Previously, the situation was very different. In the 1970s, it became apparent that patients were being infected with hepatitis viruses from the pooled clotting factor concentrates prepared from the plasma of many thousands of blood donations. Initially, hepatitis B transmission was reported, but it then became evident that many patients were being infected with a non-A, non-B virus, which was subsequently identified as hepatitis C in 1989. From the late 1970s until 1986, HIV contaminated a large proportion of clotting factor concentrates, which resulted in the infection of many patients. It became apparent that those who required the most frequent injections of concentrate (i.e. severe hemophiliacs) were at greatest risk of infection. About 60% of severe hemophiliacs in the UK and 95% of those in the USA became infected with HIV, and all patients who received concentrate also became infected with hepatitis C virus. To date, about two-thirds of those with HIV have died, but those still alive are responding well to current anti-HIV therapy with a combination of antiretroviral drugs. Of those with hepatitis C infection, about 20% have spontaneously cleared the virus, but many of the remainder have progressive chronic hepatitis which, in perhaps 20%, will lead to cirrhosis and, in some cases, to liver failure and hepatoma. Treatment with pegylated interferon and ribavirin is leading to cure in up to 50% of patients with hepatitis C infection. For those who develop end-stage cirrhosis or hepatoma, liver transplant is an option.

Combined factor V and VIII deficiency

Combined deficiency of factors V and VIII is a rare autosomal recessive bleeding disorder. Patients present with a moderate bleeding tendency, and plasma levels of factors V and VIII of 5–30 IU/dL. Recent studies have reported an association between this combined deficiency and mutations in the *LMAN1* and *CDF2* genes, which both code for proteins involved in the protein secretory pathway. It is speculated that these proteins (along with possibly another) are required for the efficient intracellular transport of factors V and VIII.

Key points – hemophilia

- Repeated hemarthroses lead to joint destruction and it is therefore important to treat every bleed early and effectively.
- Children with severe hemophilia should be treated with regular prophylactic injections of concentrate to prevent bleeding and thus preserve joint function.
- Recombinant clotting factor concentrates are preferable to those derived from plasma, because of the reduced risk of transmission of new infectious agents.
- Patients should be tested annually for the presence of inhibitors, and any patient who does not respond clinically to treatment with factor concentrate should be immediately tested for an inhibitory antibody to the therapy.
- In mild hemophilia A, desmopressin can often be effective and avoids the use of concentrate.
- All potential carriers of hemophilia A and B should be offered genetic counseling and, if appropriate, DNA testing to ascertain their carrier status.

Key references

Bowen DJ. Haemophilia A and haemophilia B: molecular insights. *Mol Pathol* 2002;55:127–44.

Hay CR, Baglin TP, Collins PW et al. The diagnosis and management of factor VIII and IX inhibitors: a guideline from the UK Haemophilia Centre Doctors' Organisation (UKHCDO). *Br J Haematol* 2000;111:78–90.

High K. Gene-based approaches to the treatment of hemophilia. *Ann N Y Acad Sci* 2002;961:63–4.

Klinge J, Ananyeva NM, Hauser CA, Saenko EL. Hemophilia A – from basic science to clinical practice. *Semin Thromb Hemost* 2002; 28:309–22.

Mannucci PM, Giangrande PL. Choice of replacement therapy for hemophilia: recombinant products only? *Hematol J* 2000;1:72–6.

Mannucci PM, Tuddenham EG. The hemophilias from royal genes to gene therapy. *N Engl J Med* 2001;344: 1773–9.

Saint-Remy JM. Immunology of factor VIII inhibitors. *Semin Thromb Hemost* 2002;28:265–8.

United Kingdom Haemophilia Centre Doctors' Organisation (UKHCDO). Guidelines on the selection and use of therapeutic products to treat haemophilia and other hereditary bleeding disorders. *Haemophilia* 2003;9:1–23.

vWD is a relatively common, usually mild, bleeding disorder caused by a reduced plasma concentration of structurally normal vWF or the presence of a structurally abnormal molecule with reduced activity. vWF is the carrier protein in plasma for factor VIII, and it also acts as a bridge between platelets and subendothelial collagen fibers.

vWF is synthesized in endothelial cells as a polypeptide of 2813 amino acids, which undergoes initial dimerization and then multimerization up to a multimer with a molecular weight (MW) of 20 million daltons. The higher MW multimers are functionally more effective in promoting platelet adhesion and aggregation. The vWF protein is released constitutively into the plasma, and is also stored in Weible–Palade bodies in the endothelial cells from which it can be released by acute exercise, desmopressin and adrenergic stimulation. vWF is also synthesized in megakaryocytes, stored in the platelet α-granules and, on activation, secreted by the platelet release reaction. This allows accumulation of vWF at the site of vascular injury where it can promote further platelet adhesion and thus hemostasis. The mature vWF protein possesses a number of specific binding sites, which represent its differing activities (Figure 7.1). Circulating high MW multimers are cleaved by a protease, known as ADAMTS-13, which is lacking in patients with the rare congenital thrombotic thrombocytopenic purpura. In vWD, the concentration of vWF is decreased and often the level of factor VIII is secondarily reduced (because without its carrier protein, it has a short plasma half-life).

Clinical features

As vWF is essential for primary hemostasis, individuals with vWD experience bruising, epistaxis, prolonged oozing from superficial cuts, menorrhagia and bleeding after trauma or surgery. Most patients present as young adults with menorrhagia or with a history of prolonged or excessive bleeding after dental surgery. vWD is usually a

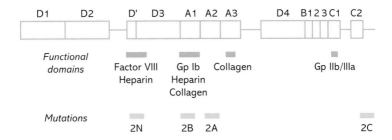

Figure 7.1 The von Willebrand factor. The protein consists of a series of domains with different binding sites for factor VIII, heparin, collagen and platelet glycoprotein (Gp) Ib and IIb/IIIa. The sites of gene mutations giving rise to different subtypes of von Willebrand's disease are marked. Reproduced courtesy of KJ Pasi.

dominantly inherited condition of variable expression and penetrance. In those with type 3 vWD (see below), inheritance is recessive, the factor VIII level is very low, and bleeding is similar to hemophilia, with hemarthroses and muscle hematoma, as well as mucosal hemorrhages.

Diagnosis

The vWF protein can be characterized by a number of different techniques, and laboratory studies reveal that there are many different phenotypic abnormalities or types of vWD.

The primary hemostatic function of vWF is best assessed by its ability to support ristocetin-induced platelet aggregation in vitro. Ristocetin was originally developed as an antibiotic, but caused thrombocytopenia when given to patients. Subsequently, it was discovered that, in the presence of vWF, ristocetin aggregated platelets and that this was dependent on the high MW multimers of vWF (which are also the most important for hemostasis).

A diagnosis of vWD requires measurement of plasma ristocetin cofactor activity, vWF antigen (together with assessment of its multimeric structure), ristocetin-induced platelet aggregation, factor VIII, platelet count and template bleeding time (Table 7.1). The

TABLE 7.1

Measurements required to diagnose and characterize von Willebrand's disease

- Factor VIII
- vWF ristocetin cofactor activity
- vWF antigen
- Ristocetin-induced platelet aggregation
- vWF multimers
- Factor VIII binding to vWF

vWF, von Willebrand factor.

diagnosis may not be straightforward as one or more of the activities of factor VIII/vWF may be borderline or even normal. It is often necessary to repeat the estimations on at least three occasions, as the concentration of both proteins is influenced by a number of endogenous factors (e.g. intercurrent illness). Both factor VIII and vWF levels are related to blood group. Those with blood group O have factor VIII/vWF levels that are 15–20% lower than those with blood group A; this should be taken into account when investigating patients with borderline results.

In some patients with normal or borderline vWF levels, a primary platelet disorder should be considered, as the clinical presentation of bleeding can be identical. In this situation, platelet function should be evaluated.

Subtypes. Of the vWD subtypes (Table 7.2), about 80% of patients have type 1 disease (quantitative reduction of a normal vWF).
- In type 2A, there is a loss of high MW multimers in some patients as a result of excessive proteolysis by ADAMTS-13.
- In type 2B, the abnormal vWF has increased affinity for platelet Gp Ib, leading to formation of platelet aggregates, which are cleared rapidly, resulting in thrombocytopenia. In this subtype, platelet aggregation is enhanced when ristocetin is added to the patient's platelet-containing plasma at low concentration (0.75 mg/mL).
- Type 2N (Normandy) is due to an abnormality at the factor VIII binding site on vWF. The condition phenotypically resembles mild

TABLE 7.2

Classification of von Willebrand's disease

Type 1	Partial quantitative deficiency of apparently normal vWF
Type 2	Qualitative deficiency of vWF
Type 2A	Qualitative variants with decreased high molecular weight multimers
Type 2B	Qualitative variants with increased affinity for platelet glycoprotein Ib
Type 2M	Qualitative variants with decreased platelet-dependent function that is not caused by the absence of high molecular weight vWF multimers
Type 2N	Qualitative variants with markedly decreased affinity for factor VIII
Type 3	Virtually complete deficiency of vWF

vWF, von Willebrand factor.
Adapted from Sadler JE. *Thromb Haemost* 1994;71:520–5.

hemophilia A, because all the commonly measured vWF activities are normal. It can only be diagnosed by measuring factor VIII binding to the patient's vWF in vitro. A further differentiating factor is that type 2N is inherited as a recessive trait, whereas inheritance is X-linked in hemophilia.

- In type 3, the level of vWF in all assays is less than 10% and factor VIII is similarly reduced, making the diagnosis straightforward in most cases.

Treatment

Treatment with desmopressin is appropriate for many patients with vWD (Tables 7.3 and 7.4). It is, therefore, usually appropriate to assess the response to a test dose (except in type 2B).

- For those with type 1 deficiency, the response to desmopressin is usually good, with a brisk rise in the level of a normally functioning vWF and factor VIII (see page 51).
- In type 2A, although the vWF level may rise in response to desmopressin, the circulating high MW molecules still undergo

rapid proteolysis and may therefore be relatively ineffective hemostatically.

- In type 2B, desmopressin, by releasing high MW multimers from endothelial cells, may induce further platelet aggregation and worsen the thrombocytopenia.
- Although desmopressin will increase the concentration of vWF in type 2N vWD, it is important to determine the duration of the beneficial effect, and particularly the duration of the elevation in factor VIII.
- In type 3, desmopressin is clinically ineffective, as any response is modest and short lived.

Treatment with a concentrate containing vWF is necessary for patients who do not respond adequately to desmopressin or in whom its use is contraindicated (Tables 7.3 and 7.4). During the manufacture of some plasma-derived factor VIII concentrates, the vWF copurifies with factor VIII and the concentrates contain both molecules. The

TABLE 7.3

Treatment of von Willebrand's disease

Classification	Treatment*
Type 1	Desmopressin; vWF concentrate if desmopressin contraindicated or for major bleed
Type 2A	vWF concentrate preferred for most bleeds; desmopressin may be adequate for minor bleed or minor surgery
Type 2B	vWF concentrate
Type 2M	vWF concentrate
Type 2N	Desmopressin (factor VIII response short-lived); vWF concentrate
Type 3	vWF concentrate

*vWF concentrates are either plasma-derived factor VIII concentrates that contain therapeutic quantities of vWF, including high MW multimers, or plasma-derived high purity vWF concentrates, which contain little factor VIII activity.
vWF, von Willebrand factor.

TABLE 7.4

Treatment doses in von Willebrand's disease

Desmopressin

- 0.3 µg/kg intravenously over 20 minutes, which can be repeated every 4–6 hours on two or three occasions
- Nasal spray administered as one application in each nostril; ensure that the concentration is 1.5 mg/mL, which is ten times the concentration used for the treatment of diabetes insipidus

vWF concentrate

- Loading dose 40–60 IU vWF/kg
- Follow-up doses every 12–24 hours to maintain vWF ristocetin cofactor activity > 0.50 IU/mL

Tranexamic acid

- Should be considered for all patients who receive desmopressin, as it inhibits the fibrinolytic response and also prevents lysis of the hemostatic plug (see Chapter 5)

vWF, von Willebrand factor.

proportion of high MW multimers in the final concentrate may be reduced and thus it is important that they contain a therapeutic level of such multimers when used to treat vWD.

After infusion of a concentrate containing vWF, responsiveness should be assessed by measuring vWF ristocetin cofactor activity and factor VIII concentration. While the level of vWF may be therapeutic (50–70 IU/dL), the factor VIII level may be in the region of 150 IU/dL, which may predispose to venous thrombosis, particularly in the postoperative period.

All currently available concentrates are derived from plasma, but as a viral inactivation step is included in their manufacture, they are very unlikely to transmit hepatitis viruses or HIV. There is still a risk, however, of parvovirus infection. All patients with vWD should be vaccinated against hepatitis A and B. Previously patients with vWD, who were treated with multiple infusions of cryoprecipitate or vWF containing factor VIII concentrates, became infected with hepatitis C or occasionally with HIV.

Key points – von Willebrand's disease

- All patients with von Willebrand's disease should be characterized by laboratory investigation as fully as possible.
- Desmopressin is effective therapy for many patients.
- When clotting factor concentrate is indicated, it should contain high molecular weight multimers of von Willebrand factor.

Key references

Allford SL, Hunt BJ, Rose P et al. Guidelines on the diagnosis and management of the thrombotic microangiopathic haemolytic anaemias. *Br J Haematol* 2003;120:556–73.

Budde U, Drewke E, Mainusch K, Schneppenheim R. Laboratory diagnosis of congenital von Willebrand disease. *Semin Thromb Hemost* 2002;28:173–90.

Favaloro EJ. Appropriate laboratory assessment as a critical facet in the proper diagnosis and classification of von Willebrand disorder. *Best Pract Res Clin Haematol* 2001;14: 299–319.

Kumar S, Pruthi RK, Nichols WL. Acquired von Willebrand disease. *Mayo Clin Proc* 2002;77:181–7.

Laffan M, Brown SA, Collins PW et al. The diagnosis of von willebrand disease: a guideline from the UK Haemophilia Centre Doctors' Organisation. *Haemophilia* 2004;10:199–217.

Pasi KJ, Collins PW, Keeling DM et al. Management of von Willebrand disease: a guideline from the UK Haemophilia Centre Doctors' Organisation. *Haemophilia* 2004;10:218–31.

Roque H, Funai E, Lockwood CJ. von Willebrand disease and pregnancy. *J Matern Fetal Med* 2000;9:257–66.

Sadler JE. Von Willebrand disease type 1: a diagnosis in search of a disease. *Blood* 2003;101:2089–93.

8 Uncommon congenital coagulation disorders

Although hemophilia A and B are the most common severe coagulation disorders, congenital deficiencies of all the other clotting factors occur and can lead to a range of clinical conditions, which may cause diagnostic and therapeutic difficulties. Most of these disorders are autosomal-recessive traits; most heterozygotes are asymptomatic, and patients are difficult to identify with clotting factor assays. Now that the technology to characterize genetic mutations is readily available, it is far more straightforward to identify heterozygotes and therefore track these disorders within families. As well as congenital disorders, acquired clotting factor deficiencies can result from an autoantibody or an alloantibody against a single clotting factor. Multiple deficiencies occur in a variety of clinical situations, but particularly in those taking oral anticoagulants, and those with liver disease or DIC (see Chapters 9–13).

Factor XI deficiency

Factor XI deficiency is inherited as an autosomal disorder, sometimes known as hemophilia C. Ashkenazi Jews are particularly affected; low levels of factor XI may be found in up to 8% of this population. Several generations within a family may have levels reduced to different degrees (Table 8.1). Individuals who are heterozygous for a mutation have a partial deficiency of factor XI, whereas those who have a severe deficiency are either homozygous or compound heterozygotes. Of the original three mutations found in affected individuals, two mutations (types 2 and 3) account for most factor XI deficiency. In type 2 deficiency, there is a stop codon in exon 5; in the homozygous state, this results in a factor XI level below 1 IU/dL. In type 3 deficiency, Phe283 is replaced with Leu (coding in exon 9); in the homozygous condition, this results in a factor XI level of approximately 10 IU/dL. A compound heterozygote of these two mutations has a factor XI level between less than 1% and 10%.

TABLE 8.1

Differences in phenotypic and genotypic expression of factor XI deficiency

In this family, only the grandfather (generation I) was known to have bleeding problems; no one in generation II or III had abnormal bleeding. The grandfather and two of the children of generation III are compound heterozygotes; the mother and father (generation II), and daughter 2 are simple heterozygotes

Generation	Mutation*	Factor XI level (% of normal)
I	2/3	< 1%
II		
Daughter of generation I	–/2	43%
Husband	–/3	66%
III		
Daughter 1	2/3	2%
Daughter 2	–/2	46%
Son	2/3	1%

*Numbers refer to mutation, either type 2, type 3 or both; –, no mutation.

Clinical features. Factor XI deficiency usually leads to excessive hemorrhage after surgery or trauma; spontaneous bleeds are rare and hemorrhages into joints and muscles uncommon.

Diagnosis. The deficiency is classified as severe if the factor XI level is less than 20 IU/dL and partial at 20–70 IU/dL; the lower limit of the normal range is 60–70 IU/dL. Unlike hemophilia A and B, the correlation between the plasma factor XI level and the propensity to bleed is poor. Individuals with similar factor XI levels may have very different hemorrhagic potential and, furthermore, this may vary over time. Bleeding usually arises following surgery, particularly dental extraction, tonsillectomy, prostatectomy and appendectomy.

Treatment. The management of bleeding and surgery in factor XI deficiency is not straightforward because of the lack of correlation between hemorrhagic potential and the plasma XI level, and because no effective and entirely safe factor XI concentrate is available. Before surgery, the postoperative bleeding risk should be assessed based on the patient's hemorrhagic history following previous surgery, the factor XI level and the severity of the impending operation.

For those with a partial deficiency, it may be appropriate to undertake surgery with only careful attention to hemostasis and to use tranexamic acid for dental extractions. For those with a severe deficiency requiring major surgery, the factor XI level may need to be raised. As the half-life of factor XI is approximately 45 hours, therapeutic infusions of plasma or concentrate are only needed once daily. Virally inactivated, fresh frozen plasma can be used, but the factor XI content of solvent/detergent-treated plasma is reduced, making this treatment relatively ineffective. An alternative is to use a factor XI concentrate. Use of these concentrates has been associated with both arterial and venous thromboembolism, and they are therefore contraindicated in those with clinical atherosclerosis and in those in whom hemostatic mechanisms are activated, such as in pregnancy and liver disease. Concentrates should not normally be used in doses above 30 IU/kg and the plasma level should not exceed 50–70 IU/dL. Fibrinolytic inhibitors should never be given concomitantly with a factor XI concentrate, because of their propensity to predispose to thrombosis and DIC. Patients with the type 2 defect often develop inhibitory antibodies when exposed to normal factor XI. Such antibodies may induce resistance to further treatment with factor XI, and call for the use of activated prothrombin complex concentrate or recombinant activated human factor VIIa for the control of bleeding.

Factor VII deficiency

Congenital factor VII deficiency is an uncommon autosomal recessive disorder whose prevalence is much higher in countries where consanguineous marriages are common. The correlation between bleeding risk and factor VII level is poor. Individuals with a moderate factor VII deficiency often bleed from the mucous membranes, and epistaxis, bleeding gums and menorrhagia are common. In severe factor VII deficiency, bleeding into the central nervous system (CNS) very early in life leads to a high morbidity and mortality. Hemarthroses have been reported in severe factor VII deficiency but, unlike in hemophilia A and B, are not a common feature.

The most common causes of factor VII deficiency are acquired, and include liver disease and ingestion of a vitamin K antagonist oral anticoagulant (e.g. warfarin; see Chapter 13). In liver disease, the level of factor VII is used as a measure of the degree of hepatic dysfunction. Rarely, a deficiency is observed in patients taking penicillins or cephalosporins, and it has also been reported in patients with myeloma or sepsis.

Diagnosis. Congenital factor VII deficiency is usually suspected when an isolated prolongation of the PT is found in a patient without liver disease, and a normal APTT and normal fibrinogen level. In some cases, the apparent level of factor VII varies with the source of thromboplastin used for the PT test.

Treatment. The treatment of choice is recombinant human factor VIIa concentrate, but virally inactivated fresh frozen plasma, prothrombin complex concentrate (containing factors II, VII, IX and X) and plasma-derived factor VII concentrate can be used to treat acute bleeds or cover surgery. As the half-life of factor VII in vivo is about 5 hours, repeated and frequent infusions are needed.

Factor X deficiency

Congenital factor X deficiency is a rare autosomal-recessive disorder, and many patients with symptomatic bleeding are homozygous, though a few double heterozygotes have been reported. The differential diagnosis includes acquired factor X deficiency resulting from either warfarin therapy or liver disease when it is accompanied by a reduction in the level of other clotting factors. Isolated acquired factor X deficiency is occasionally found in association with other disorders, particularly amyloidosis; in this condition, the circulating factor X is rapidly cleared from the circulation by binding to the amyloid protein.

Clinical features. The bleeding manifestations are very similar to those of factor VII deficiency.

Treatment can be with either virally inactivated fresh frozen plasma or prothrombin complex concentrate. As the half-life of factor X is 24–40 hours, a single daily infusion is usually adequate. A factor X level of 10–40 IU/dL is usually considered hemostatic.

Factor II deficiency

Congenital deficiencies of factor II (prothrombin) are due to homozygous or double heterozygous genetic mutations and are, therefore, recessively inherited. Bleeding manifestations are similar to those with deficiencies of factors VII and X. Treatment is with fresh frozen plasma or prothrombin complex concentrate.

Combined deficiencies of factors II, VII, IX and X

Rarely, a congenital combined deficiency of factors II, VII, IX and X, as well as proteins C and S, is seen. It is caused by deficiency of vitamin K dependent carboxylase as a result of homozygous genetic mutations. This condition must be distinguished from acquired deficiencies caused by liver disease or warfarin. Treatment with oral vitamin K increases the plasma level of these clotting factors, and fresh frozen plasma or prothrombin complex concentrate are effective for acute bleeds.

Factor V deficiency

Congenital factor V deficiency is a rare, recessively inherited disorder. Besides its presence in plasma, factor V is also stored and secreted from platelet α-granules during the release reaction that occurs during formation of the hemostatic plug. It has been suggested that the level of factor V in platelets is a better reflection of the bleeding potential than the plasma concentration. Patients bleed from the mucous membranes and also into the CNS. Treatment is with fresh frozen plasma as there is no concentrate containing factor V; platelet transfusions may also be effective.

Fibrinogen deficiency

The hypo- and dysfibrinogenemias comprise a collection of disorders that are usually dominantly inherited and associated with both bleeding and venous thrombotic manifestations.

Clinical features. Bleeding usually arises following trauma or surgery, presents as placental abruption or occurs postpartum. Venous thromboembolism may also be observed in association with pregnancy or in other clinical situations of increased risk.

Treatment is with a virally inactivated, plasma-derived fibrinogen concentrate. The half-life of fibrinogen is about 5 days, and therefore infusions usually only need to be given every 2–3 days. The trough plasma fibrinogen level should be kept above 1.0 g/L, and many advocate maintaining it above 1.5 g/L.

Factor XIII deficiency

Congenital deficiency of factor XIII is a rare autosomal-recessive disorder. It is characterized by features of delayed and impaired wound healing with bleeding often occurring 24–36 hours after surgery or trauma. Bleeding from the umbilical stump is common, and soft tissue bleeds, including muscle hematoma, are more common than hemarthroses, which only occur after trauma. Spontaneous intracranial bleeds are also a characteristic feature, and are the principal cause of morbidity and mortality. Spontaneous abortion in early pregnancy is also typical. The severity of the bleeding state varies markedly between individuals with apparently similar factor XIII plasma levels.

Treatment. Factor XIII has a long half-life of about 11 days and, as it is only necessary to keep the level above about 2% of normal to prevent spontaneous bleeds, a single infusion may be required only every 4 weeks. Therapy should be with a virally inactivated, plasma-derived factor XIII concentrate. Because of the risk of intracranial hemorrhage in particular, it is customary to treat patients with monthly prophylactic infusions, which are effective in preventing almost all spontaneous bleeds.

Key points – uncommon congenital coagulation disorders

Factor XI deficiency
- Family members should be fully investigated for both factor XI clotting activity and the mutation(s) in the gene, because compound heterozygotes are common.
- Unlike in hemophilia A, the level of factor XI is not a good predictor of bleeding risk.
- Factor XI concentrates should be used with caution, because they predispose to arterial and venous thromboembolism. Fresh frozen plasma is often effective therapy, but exposure to normal factor XI in plasma or concentrates carries a risk of inhibitor development in those with type 2 disease.

Factor VII deficiency
- Bleeding is uncommon in factor VII heterozygotes.
- Individuals with severe factor VII deficiency are usually homozygous and originate from consanguineous marriages.
- In severe factor VII deficiency, bleeding can be common and severe, including intracranial hemorrhage. Treatment with recombinant human factor VIIa is effective.

Fibrinogen deficiency
- Congenital hypofibrinogenemia predisposes to venous thromboembolism, postoperative and postpartum hemorrhage, and placental abruption.
- As fibrinogen has a long half-life of 5 days, effective prophylactic therapy can be given readily to cover surgery and throughout pregnancy.

Key references

Asakai R, Chung DW, Ratnoff OD, Davie EW. Factor XI deficiency in Ashkenazi Jews is a bleeding disorder that can result from three types of point mutations. *Proc Natl Acad Sci U S A* 1989;86:7667–71.

Bolton Maggs PHB. Factor XI deficiency and its management. *Haemophilia* 2000;6(suppl 1);100–9.

Brennan SO, Fellowes AP, George PM. Molecular mechanisms of hypo- and afibrinogenemia. *Ann N Y Acad Sci* 2001;936:91–100.

Ichinose A. Physiopathology and regulation of factor XIII. *Thromb Haemost* 2001;86:57–65.

Kato H. Regulation of functions of vascular wall cells by tissue factor pathway inhibitor: basic and clinical aspects. *Arterioscler Thromb Vasc Biol* 2002;22:539–48.

Lorand L. Factor XIII: structure, activation, and interactions with fibrinogen and fibrin. *Ann N Y Acad Sci* 2001;936:291–311.

Neerman-Arbez M. The molecular basis of inherited afibrinogenaemia. *Thromb Haemost* 2001;86:154–63.

Perry D. Factor VII deficiency. *Br J Haematol* 2002;118:689.

Roberts HR, Stinchcombe TE, Gabriel DA. The dysfibrinogenaemias. *Br J Haematol* 2001;114:249–57.

Salomon O, Zivelin A, Livnat T et al. Prevalence, causes, and characterization of factor XI inhibitors in patients with inherited factor XI deficiency. *Blood* 2003;101:4783–8.

Liver disorders

The coagulation changes in patients with liver disease are complex and often arise as a result of several different mechanisms. The liver is the principal site for synthesis and also clearance of many of the coagulant and fibrinolytic proteins. In many instances, the coagulopathy results from a combination of decreased synthesis and shortened half-life of the hemostatic components. A variety of mechanisms cause the coagulation changes that are discussed below, but many can be attributed to cytokine activation, particularly increased production of TNFα. The complexity of the situation is further compounded by the fact that the liver is made up of three cell types (hepatocytes, Kupffer cells and endothelial cells), each with very different characteristics and functions. The bleeding risk is also dependent on the platelet count, which is influenced by the degree of splenomegaly secondary to liver-induced portal hypertension. In the absence of liver disease, portal hypertension is also observed in hepatic venous thrombosis (Budd–Chiari syndrome), and in portal or splenic venous thrombosis.

The coagulation changes depend on the pathogenesis of the underlying liver disease and its rate of onset. In general, liver disease can be divided, from the perspective of hemostasis, into the following four broad groups:

- acute hepatitis characterized predominantly by a consumptive coagulopathy
- cirrhosis in which there is decreased synthesis of clotting factors
- biliary obstruction, which leads to vitamin K deficiency
- tumors, which arise in cirrhosis and are particularly associated with dysfibrinogenemia.

Some of the hemostatic abnormalities that contribute to the coagulopathy are discussed below.

Decreased synthesis of clotting factors. Chronic liver disease, such as cirrhosis, results in diminished synthesis of clotting factors, especially factors II, VII, IX and X. As factor VII has the shortest half-life (about 5 hours), its level is often the lowest. The PT is most sensitive to factor VII deficiency and is therefore useful in assessing the synthetic capacity of the liver.

Impaired γ-carboxylation of factors II, VII, IX and X. Carboxylation of the inactive peptides for factors II, VII, IX and X by hepatocyte γ-carboxylase results in their conversion to clotting factors that can participate in hemostasis. In chronic liver disease, carboxylase activity is reduced and, as a result, carboxylation of the precursor peptides is incomplete. Furthermore, the carboxylation process depends on vitamin K; if vitamin K is lacking (e.g. in biliary obstruction), clotting factor levels, particularly factor VII, may underestimate the true capacity of the liver for synthesis. Therefore, before using the PT to assess liver function, it may be prudent to give parenteral vitamin K, 10 mg diluted in 50 mL saline, by slow intravenous infusion.

Fibrinogen. The liver has a large capacity to synthesize fibrinogen and the plasma level is maintained until late in liver failure. By the time the level falls below 1 g/L, there is usually severe fulminant disease or end-stage decompensated cirrhosis. If infection is present, the fibrinogen level may be reduced more than would be expected for the degree of hepatic impairment as a result of the consumptive coagulopathy of DIC. On the other hand, in the inflammation that accompanies some forms of chronic hepatitis (e.g. biliary cirrhosis), the increased level of TNFα promotes the increased synthesis of fibrinogen and consequently raises the plasma level.

Fibrinolysis. A variety of changes in fibrinolysis are observed in liver disease. In acute hepatitis and cirrhosis, primary fibrinolysis results from reduced clearance of tPA by the diseased liver. Fibrinolysis may also be impaired by increased synthesis of PAI-1 or diminished synthesis of plasminogen; conversely, it may be enhanced by impaired production of α_2-antiplasmin. Secondary fibrinolysis may be observed with DIC that may accompany septicemia or fulminant hepatic failure, and may be mediated by TNFα secretion by hepatic Kupffer or other reticuloendothelial cells.

Factors VIII and V. Factor VIII is produced by endothelial cells as well as being synthesized in the liver. In hepatic disease, therefore, its synthesis is not just dependent on the capacity of hepatocyte function. In cirrhosis, the factor VIII level is often normal, but in inflammatory as well as acute hepatitis, the plasma factor VIII level may be markedly raised, probably as a result of the secretion of the cytokine interleukin (IL)-6. A feature of DIC is a reduced level of factor VIII due to its consumption in the intravascular coagulative process.

Factor V is also synthesized predominantly by the liver; a reduced plasma level is a feature of liver failure. Like factor VIII, factor V can be consumed in DIC, resulting in lower levels than would be anticipated for the degree of liver failure. It is sometimes useful to measure factors V and VIII to distinguish the coagulopathy of DIC from that of liver disease. In DIC, levels of both factors are decreased, whereas in liver disease, factor V is low, but factor VIII is usually normal or high.

Platelets. In liver disease, the platelet count is usually normal or reduced. The liver is a source of thrombopoietin, a protein that stimulates platelet production; decreased concentrations have been reported in patients with liver failure. Mild splenomegaly results in platelet pooling and a platelet count in the range $75–125 \times 10^9/L$ often accompanies cirrhosis. The count may be further reduced by alcohol intake, which inhibits the production of platelets by megakaryocytes. Stopping alcohol consumption often results in a sharp rise in the platelet count after several days. Folate deficiency, which may accompany alcoholic cirrhosis, will exacerbate any thrombocytopenia and can be remedied by folic acid supplementation. Reduced platelet function (e.g. impaired aggregation to ADP) may be seen in some patients and may contribute to the bleeding severity.

Coagulation inhibitors. Impaired antithrombin synthesis in the diseased liver leads to a reduced plasma concentration, which may predispose to a consumptive coagulopathy. The anticoagulants, proteins C and S, are both vitamin K dependent, and their carboxylation and thus function is impaired in cirrhosis. These prothrombotic changes are usually balanced by the anticoagulant effects of the other changes in severe liver disease described above.

Disseminated intravascular coagulation. Patients with both advanced liver disease and severe acute hepatitis are at risk of DIC (see Chapter 12). The precipitating event may be Gram-negative septicemia caused by impaired clearance of bacteria that gain entry to the portal system from the gut or another source of infection (e.g. ascites). The diagnosis of DIC can be difficult, because it arises in the setting of some of the disturbances of clotting described above, but with careful investigation it is often possible to establish the predominant cause of the coagulation changes.

Diagnosis. Initial investigations comprise a full blood count and a coagulation screen consisting of APTT, PT, fibrinogen and D-dimer (a measure of FDPs). The typical patterns of abnormalities associated with the different mechanisms are given in Table 9.1. In patients in whom it is unclear whether the coagulation changes are due to severe liver disease or DIC, measurement of factors VII and VIII may helpful, as a reduction in factor VII suggests severe impairment of synthesis and a reduction in factor VIII suggests DIC.

TABLE 9.1

Typical patterns of abnormalities associated with liver disease

	Platelets	APTT	PT	Factor V	Factor VII	Fibrinogen
Acute hepatitis						
Without liver failure	N	N	N or ↑	N or ↓	N or ↓	N or ↑
With liver failure	N or ↓	↑	↑↑	↓↓	↓↓	↓↓
Liver cirrhosis	N or ↓	N or ↑	↑	↓ or N	↓	N or ↓
Biliary obstruction	N	↑ or N	↑↑	N or ↑	↓↓	↑ or N

APTT, activated partial thromboplastin time; PT, prothrombin time; N, normal; ↑, increased; ↓, decreased.

Treatment of the coagulopathy associated with liver disease is necessary for patients with active bleeding or who are about to undergo an invasive procedure (e.g. liver biopsy). It is important to be satisfied that the patient does not have a vitamin K deficiency; if there is any doubt, vitamin K_1, 10 mg diluted in 50 mL saline, should be administered cautiously by intravenous infusion, and the coagulation tests repeated after 12 hours. Fresh frozen plasma, 20 mL/kg, is the most commonly used therapy to increase coagulation factor levels. It is not, however, particularly effective; the increase in concentrations is short-lived, and the treatment cannot readily be repeated because of the large volume of plasma that needs to be given. Cryoprecipitate is a good source of fibrinogen; 5–10 bags will usually increase fibrinogen levels by at least 1 g/L. Prothrombin concentrates containing factors II, VII, IX and X increase levels of these clotting factors effectively, but they carry a risk of precipitating thrombosis and DIC, particularly in those with advanced liver disease, and are therefore rarely used. For patients with DIC, antithrombin concentrate may improve the coagulopathy, but there is no evidence that it improves the prognosis.

Occasionally, heparin therapy is used to reduce the severity of DIC, but this is of unproven value and is potentially unwise in a patient with esophageal varices or gastritis. Very occasionally, a fibrinolytic inhibitor (e.g. tranexamic acid) may be used if diffuse bleeding is due to excessive fibrinolysis, but it also potentially predisposes to thrombosis or excessive fibrin deposition, which could impair organ function (e.g. induce renal failure).

Thrombocytopenia can be treated with platelet transfusion. The transfusion should be given immediately before a procedure, because the platelets quickly become pooled in the enlarged spleen. The platelet count needs to be at least 50×10^9/L for even minor surgery, but many would recommend a level of 70–80×10^9/L.

Kidney disorders

The bleeding observed in patients with renal failure, usually bruising and gastrointestinal hemorrhage, has many of the features of a disorder of primary hemostasis, but the abnormality is in the platelet–vessel wall interaction. In most patients, no abnormality can be detected in the coagulation mechanism. Dialysis substantially reduces the risk of bleeding and is the mainstay of management to keep the hemorrhagic risk under control.

Etiology of hemorrhagic state. In renal failure, the most consistent abnormality is a prolongation of the bleeding time that correlates with the bleeding symptoms, but not with the plasma urea or creatinine level. The platelet count is usually normal or mildly reduced, and thrombocytopenia does not contribute to prolongation of the bleeding time. The results of platelet aggregation tests are extremely variable and are not related to bleeding risk. A number of possible mechanisms contribute to the bleeding risk (Table 9.2).

Accumulation of dialyzable uremic toxins impairs primary hemostasis; potential candidates include urea, guanidinosuccinic acid and phenols, which inhibit platelet aggregation. It has been hypothesized that other dialyzable substances stimulate endothelial production of prostacyclin and nitric oxide, which inhibit platelet

TABLE 9.2

Mechanisms contributing to defective hemostasis in uremia

Platelet function defects

- Decreased aggregation
- Increased cAMP and cGMP
- Decreased thromboxane production

Endothelial cell defects

- Increased synthesis and release of prostacyclin and nitric oxide

Vessel wall platelet defects

- Diminished platelet adhesion
- Reduced von Willebrand factor activity

Anemia

cAMP, cyclic adenosine monophosphate; cGMP, cyclic guanosine monophosphate.

adenyl cyclase and guanidyl cyclase. This leads to an increase in the intracellular concentration of platelet inhibitory cyclic adenosine monophosphate (cAMP) and cyclic guanosine monophosphate (cGMP), respectively. Parathormone is elevated in renal failure and also increases platelet cAMP.

Intrinsic platelet defects include decreased ADP and serotonin in the platelet dense granules. Reduced platelet aggregation may be due to depressed platelet production of the potent platelet agonist thromboxane A$_2$.

vWF abnormalities may impair adhesion of platelets to the vessel wall.

Anemia contributes to the bleeding risk; there is an inverse relationship between the bleeding time and hematocrit. Raising the hemoglobin level improves hemostasis, probably by increasing the margination of platelets to the damaged vessel wall. More ADP is released from the red cells, which promotes platelet aggregation and the formation of the hemostatic plug. The hematocrit needs to be raised to 27–32% to normalize the bleeding time.

Clinical features of uremic bleeding. Bleeding is predominantly into the skin and mucous membranes; purpura, ecchymoses, epistaxis, upper gastrointestinal bleeding and hemorrhagic pericarditis are common. Retroperitoneal bleeding can occur and may arise as a complication of femoral catheterization for hemodialysis. Some patients with renal failure are also prone to thrombosis, including repeated clotting of shunts, and arterial and venous thromboembolism. Accelerated atherosclerosis is also a feature of renal failure, possibly because the release of platelet-derived growth factor induces smooth muscle proliferation in the vessel wall, or as a result of endothelial injury from hyperhomocysteinemia.

Treatment of bleeding

Dialysis. Both hemodialysis and peritoneal dialysis generally reduce the bleeding risk, though they may not be equally effective in all patients. The effect of dialysis on the normalization of bleeding time and platelet aggregation is variable.

> **Key points – liver and kidney disorders**
>
> Liver disorders
> - Acute and chronic liver disease can give rise to a variety of different hemostatic disorders; it is therefore important to assess each patient fully.
> - Vitamin K therapy should be given if there is any possibility of deficiency of this vitamin.
> - Although many patients have abnormal clotting tests, it is usually only necessary to treat those patients who are actively bleeding or require surgical intervention.
>
> Kidney disorders
> - The risk of bleeding increases with the degree of renal failure.
> - Dialysis reduces the hemorrhagic risk.
> - Correction of anemia in the short term by red cell transfusion or in the long term with regular erythropoietin injections reduces the risk of bleeding.

Correction of anemia. Together with dialysis, correction of the anemia is a mainstay of treatment to reduce the hemorrhagic risk. Regular red cell transfusions are effective in controlling hemostasis, but the accumulation of iron and the risk of acquiring infection make this approach unattractive. Recombinant erythropoietin, 150–300 U/kg/week, raises the hematocrit effectively. The hematocrit should be increased to 27–32% because, at this level, the bleeding time becomes normal, but the risks of hypertension, encephalopathy, thrombosis and hyperkalemia, which arise if the hematocrit is rapidly raised to 40% or above, are avoided.

Cryoprecipitate. An infusion of cryoprecipitate shortens the bleeding time for about 24–36 hours, and bleeding often ceases. The beneficial effect is attributed to the vWF content of the cryoprecipitate.

Desmopressin. High MW vWF multimers are released from endothelial cells by desmopressin (see page 50). In patients with renal failure, desmopressin shortens the bleeding time and improves hemostasis. Repeated infusions result in tachyphylaxis, but two or three injections of 0.3 µg/kg intravenously or subcutaneously at 4–8-hour intervals can be effective. Desmopressin can also be administered intranasally at a dose of 300 µg (150 µg in each nostril).

Key references

Amitrano L, Guardascione MA, Brancaccio V, Balzano A. Coagulation disorders in liver disease. *Semin Liver Dis* 2002; 22:83–96.

Kuter DJ, Begley CG. Recombinant human thrombopoietin: basic biology and evaluation of clinical studies. *Blood* 2002;100:3457–69.

McCormick PA, Murphy KM. Splenomegaly, hypersplenism and coagulation abnormalities in liver disease. *Baillieres Best Pract Res Clin Gastroenterol* 2000;14:1009–31.

Opatrny K Jr. Hemostasis disorders in chronic renal failure. *Kidney Int Suppl* 1997;62:S87–9.

Ozier Y, Steib A, Ickx B et al. Haemostatic disorders during liver transplantation. *Eur J Anaesthesiol* 2001;18:208–18.

Rapaport SI. Coagulation problems in liver disease. *Blood Coagul Fibrinolysis* 2000;11(suppl 1): S69–74.

Schetz MR. Coagulation disorders in acute renal failure. *Kidney Int Suppl* 1998;66:S96–101.

Tang WW, Stead RA, Goodkin DA. Effects of epoetin alfa on hemostasis in chronic renal failure. *Am J Nephrol* 1998;18:263–73.

During normal pregnancy, a series of progressive changes in hemostasis occur that are procoagulant and help prevent excessive hemorrhage at the time of delivery. This tilting of the balance to protect against bleeding, however, results in a marked increase in thrombotic risk. The incidence of venous thromboembolism increases about fourfold during normal pregnancy and is greatest in the puerperium.

The plasma concentrations of coagulation factors VII, VIII, X, vWF and fibrinogen start to increase during the first trimester and, by the end of pregnancy, may have increased by 50–100%. Fibrinolysis becomes increasingly inhibited, not only by the rise in PAI-1, but also by PAI-2, which is secreted in increasing amounts by the placenta. The concentration of its cofactor, free protein S (but not protein C), declines by up to 50% of that in the non-pregnant state, thereby reducing the anticoagulant activity of the protein C/S pathway.

The platelet count declines by 10% in pregnancy, partly as a result of the increase in plasma volume.

Gestational thrombocytopenia

Although the platelet count declines in normal pregnancy, a fall below the lower limit of normal (150×10^9/L) is uncommon. In about 10% of pregnancies, however, it falls to $100–150 \times 10^9$/L without any coagulation disturbance or presence of other illness. This gestational or 'benign' thrombocytopenia of pregnancy is of unknown etiology and is of no clinical consequence. Babies born to mothers with this disorder have normal platelet counts. It is an entirely benign condition and the skill is to exclude other causes of thrombocytopenia and make a positive diagnosis. It is usually necessary to monitor the platelet count because, if it falls below 100×10^9/L, the diagnosis must be reviewed.

Immune thrombocytopenic purpura (ITP)

ITP is a relatively common cause of isolated thrombocytopenia due to the presence of an antiplatelet antibody in the plasma (see page 111). It is usually diagnosed by excluding other causes of a reduced platelet count (e.g. DIC). Preexisting ITP may be exacerbated during pregnancy, and the platelet count declines further to a level at which specific treatment may be required. ITP may also first present in pregnancy with a platelet count of less than 100×10^9/L on routine blood examination, or with bleeding symptoms, which usually only occur when the platelet count is less than 20×10^9/L. As in the non-pregnant state, it is important to exclude other causes of thrombocytopenia (see Chapter 4) and, in particular, to ensure that the patient does not have a primary bone marrow disorder (e.g. acute leukemia).

If the platelet count falls below about 30×10^9/L, prednisone, 0.5–1.0 mg/kg, should be started and the response monitored. It may be necessary to increase the dose or give intravenous immunoglobulin, 0.4 g/kg/day for 5 days or 1 g/kg/day for 2 days, to maintain the platelet count above 30×10^9/L. Anti-rhesus D immunoglobulin 50–100 µg/kg is an alternative that is currently being examined in clinical trials for women who are rhesus positive and who have not undergone splenectomy.

The antiplatelet antibody responsible for the ITP may cross the placenta; the cord blood platelet count of all babies born to mothers with this condition should therefore be checked. The incidence of thrombocytopenia at birth is 10–50% and is usually mild, though the platelet count can drop further in the first few days of life. It is therefore prudent to recheck the count after a few days. It is not possible to predict the cord blood platelet count in advance of delivery. The risk of fetal bleeding during labor is extremely small, even with severe thrombocytopenia, and it is therefore inappropriate to obtain an antenatal platelet count by fetal blood sampling before or during labor. Furthermore, cesarean section does not appear to offer any greater protection to the neonate than an uncomplicated vaginal delivery. The use of forceps, however, should be avoided.

Neonatal alloimmune thrombocytopenia

Neonatal alloimmune thrombocytopenia (NAIT) is an uncommon condition in which maternal immunization occurs to a platelet antigen present on fetal and the paternal, but not maternal, platelets.

Transplacental transfer of the antiplatelet IgG reacts with the fetal platelets and causes severe thrombocytopenia. NAIT is analogous to red cell rhesus hemolytic disease of the newborn. It usually arises in mothers who do not possess the platelet antigen HPA-1A, which is found in 97% of the population, and who have a fetus that is HPA-IA positive. Minor feto-maternal bleeds across the placenta lead to the development of maternal anti-HPA-1A. NAIT is often associated with intracranial hemorrhage in the fetus during gestation or at delivery.

Management of subsequent pregnancies requires determination of whether the father is heterozygous for HPA-1A and, if so, whether a fetus in a subsequent pregnancy might possess this antigen. If the fetus would have the antigen, there is a high risk of recurrence. Possible interventions include intrauterine transfusions of maternal HPA-1A negative platelets.

Pregnancy-induced hypertension

Hypertension, proteinuria and edema characterize pregnancy-induced hypertension (PIH), which is most common in primigravidas. One of the other features of PIH is activation of the coagulation system and thrombocytopenia possibly arising secondary to endothelial damage. There is deposition of fibrin in the placenta and, in its more severe form, DIC and a generalized consumptive coagulopathy.

Following delivery of the fetus, the features of PIH resolve quickly. Induction of labor may, therefore, be appropriate in late pregnancy if PIH is severe and unresponsive to medical management. If the DIC is severe with a fibrinogen level of less than 1 g/L and platelets less than 50×10^9/L, it may be necessary to give blood products (see DIC below).

HELLP syndrome is seen in a small percentage of patients with PIH and is characterized by hemolysis, elevated liver enzymes and low platelets. The hemolysis is usually mild, but fragmented erythrocytes are present on the peripheral blood smear and the level of LDH is elevated, as are hepatic enzymes (e.g. alanine aminotransferase).

Disseminated intravascular coagulation

Clinical presentation. The activated coagulation system in pregnancy reduces the threshold for DIC. Conditions causing the consumptive coagulopathy are listed in Table 10.1. Clinically, the patient may present with:

- a trigger, such as placental abruption or amniotic fluid embolism
- the hemorrhagic and cardiovascular complications of DIC (e.g. ecchymoses, hematuria and shock)
- thrombotic complications in the brain, kidney or lung.

Diagnosis. A fibrinogen level lower than would be expected for the gestational period is diagnostic. The fibrinogen level rises progressively during pregnancy and may be 4–6 g/L by delivery. Thus, a fibrinogen level within the normal adult non-pregnant range (1.5–4.0 g/L) is relatively reduced for the stage of gestation.

Management. The precipitating cause should be eliminated as quickly as possible. If the patient is bleeding, it is necessary to give appropriate blood products in an attempt to restore coagulation and platelet count (see page 106). In the absence of hemorrhage, blood products, such as cryoprecipitate, are only necessary if the fibrinogen level is less than 1 g/L and the platelet count less than 50×10^9/L to cover delivery.

TABLE 10.1

Obstetric causes of disseminated intravascular coagulation

- Placental abruption
- Preeclampsia/HELLP syndrome of pregnancy
- Major hemorrhage
- Septic and induced abortion
- Intrauterine fetal death
- Amniotic fluid embolism
- Acute fatty liver of pregnancy

HELLP, hemolytic anemia with elevated liver enzymes and low platelets.

Placental abruption is the most common cause of severe DIC. A large retroplacental hematoma develops with extensive deposition of fibrin and platelets, leading to thrombocytopenia and hypofibrinogenemia. Urgent cesarean section is required to save the fetus, and limit the hemorrhage and coagulopathy. Amniotic fluid embolization is a catastrophic event characterized by sudden, severe dyspnea, hypotension and bleeding. Acute pulmonary hypertension occurs and fetal squames and hair, for example, are discovered in the pulmonary alveoli. Urgent resuscitative measures including ventilatory support and blood products are required.

Retention of a dead fetus will, after several weeks, lead to DIC because of the release of thromboplastin, which activates coagulation. The coagulopathy can sometimes be managed by giving intravenous heparin that interrupts the consumptive process. It may take several days for coagulation to return to normal to allow evacuation of the uterus.

TABLE 10.2

Causes of obstetric hemorrhage

Placenta

- Placenta previa
- Placental abruption
- Placental vessels
- Retained products of conception

Uterus

- Cesarean section
- Placental bed
- Placenta acreata
- Uterine atonia

Cervix and vagina

- Trauma at delivery

Obstetric hemorrhage

Major obstetric hemorrhage is life threatening; the causes are listed
in Table 10.2. Once major bleeding is revealed or suspected, prompt
intervention is required with intravenous fluid and red cells, together
with fresh frozen plasma and platelets if coagulopathy is present.
Furthermore, the underlying cause must be attended to immediately
(e.g. retained placenta). Once more than 10 units of packed red cells
have been given, it is likely that platelets and fresh frozen plasma
will be required, because a dilutional coagulopathy is likely to
have developed.

Key points – pregnancy

- In pregnancy, it is important to be aware of the complications
  that may be associated with severe coagulation disturbance
  (e.g. pregnancy-associated hypertension), and to monitor the
  blood count and coagulation screen in these patients.
- Before attributing a platelet count of 100×10^9/L or less to the
  benign condition of gestational thrombocytopenia of
  pregnancy, other causes of a reduced platelet count should be
  excluded.
- In immune thrombocytopenic purpura, the platelet count tends
  to fall as pregnancy progresses and treatment may be necessary
  to maintain it above about 50×10^9/L. After delivery, the
  platelet count in the neonate should be monitored for about a
  week as it can fall profoundly in the first few days of life.

Key reference

Williams MD, Chalmers EA,
Gibson BE et al. The investigation
and management of neonatal
haemostasis and thrombosis. *Br J
Haematol* 2002;119:295–309.

11

Preoperative assessment

Nothing makes a surgeon happier than the knowledge that a patient does not have a bleeding tendency. Many laboratory tests have been developed to provide the surgeon with that assurance, but unfortunately none is as reliable as a carefully taken medical history. The normal hemostatic mechanism and routine assessment tests are discussed in Chapter 2; however, a normal coagulation screen does not exclude a bleeding disorder.

History. Important clinical clues to a bleeding tendency are:
- previous spontaneous bleeding, such as nosebleeds that are not easily controllable with external pressure, and spontaneous bruising, especially on the trunk
- excessive bleeding with previous surgery or dental extractions; for example, a need to return to the dentist because of recurrent bleeding from the socket
- menorrhagia, defined as excessive bleeding beyond the usual first 48 hours of menses, bleeding persisting for more than 5–7 days, or a history of blood-loss anemia
- the use of medications, such as aspirin, clopidogrel, oral anticoagulants, NSAIDs or herbal agents (Table 11.1)
- a family history of bleeding.

Examination. The physical findings that suggest a possible bleeding disorder are:
- skin – petechiae, purpura, bruises, telangiectasias, wide scars and hyperelasticity
- abdominal organs – enlargement of the liver or spleen
- muscles and joints – hematomas, hemarthroses or chronic large joint arthropathy.

Laboratory testing should mainly be used to investigate clinical impressions. If the history and physical examination do not suggest a

TABLE 11.1

Herbal medications to avoid before surgery*

Medication	How long to avoid before surgery	Potential adverse effect
Garlic	7 days	Bleeding risk
Ginkgo	36 hours	Bleeding risk
Ginseng	7 days	Bleeding and low blood sugar
Ephedra	24 hours	Heart attack and stroke
Echinacea	As long as possible	Allergic reactions, immune suppression
St John's wort	5 days	Increased metabolism of many drugs used in the perioperative period

*Data from Ang-Lee M. *JAMA* 2001;286:208–16.

bleeding disorder, laboratory studies are unlikely to be helpful. Often, extensive laboratory testing yields borderline abnormalities that do not predict bleeding and merely waste time. On the other hand, laboratory tests may be normal in patients with a clear history of previous bleeding; usually these patients have excessive surgical blood loss despite the normal tests. It is only when the history and the laboratory tests are congruent that an accurate diagnosis can be established, and appropriate measures implemented to avoid perioperative bleeding.

Investigations. A history of bleeding from mucous membranes in the mouth, nose and gastrointestinal or genitourinary tracts suggests either a platelet disorder or vWD. Appropriate tests in such cases are a platelet count and a measure of platelet function, either the bleeding time or the platelet function analyzer (PFA)-100 (Table 11.2). The bleeding time test is described in Figure 2.3 on page 21. The PFA-100 applies a citrated blood sample to a collagen-coated membrane containing a 150 μm aperture, in the presence of either epinephrine or ADP. The time required for complete occlusion of the aperture is recorded.

TABLE 11.2

Comparison of the bleeding time test and the platelet function analyzer (PFA)-100

	Bleeding time	PFA-100
Abnormalities detected	• Decreased platelet count • Effect of drugs, such as aspirin and NSAIDs • von Willebrand's disease • Low hematocrit • Renal failure • Vasculitis, amyloidosis, scurvy	• Decreased platelet count • Aspirin, NSAIDs detected by adrenaline (epinephrine) reagent • von Willebrand's disease, sickle cell disease • Low hematocrit • Renal failure
Invasive	Possible skin scarring	Venepuncture only
Requires technical expertise	Yes	No
Cost of equipment	Inexpensive	Expensive
Availability	Usually only daytime	24 hours if equipment available

NSAIDs, non-steroidal anti-inflammatory drugs.

If these tests are normal, bleeding due to a platelet disorder is unlikely, but more sophisticated tests are needed to exclude vWD, since the bleeding time and PFA-100 are not always abnormal in this condition (see Chapter 7).

Patients with a history of bleeding after surgery or trauma may have hemophilia or liver disease, which can be diagnosed by measurement of the APPT and PT (Table 11.3). If the patient has a strong history suggestive of a bleeding disorder with normal screening tests, specific clotting factor levels should be measured or more detailed tests of platelet function performed.

A prolonged APTT with a normal PT is usually observed in patients receiving heparin, or when heparin contaminates a line being used for

TABLE 11.3

Interpretation of activated partial thromboplastin time (APTT) and prothrombin time (PT) results

APTT prolonged, PT normal	PT prolonged, APTT normal	Both APTT and PT prolonged
• Low factors XII, XI, IX and VIII	• Low factor VII	• Low factors I, II, V and X
• Lupus anticoagulant	• Liver disease	• Liver disease (late)
• Heparin	• Vitamin K deficiency (early)	• Vitamin K deficiency (late)
• Low prekallikrein	• Warfarin (within first 2 weeks of initiation)	• Warfarin (after 2 weeks of therapy)
• Low high molecular weight kininogen		• High hematocrit

blood sampling. The presence of heparin may be readily suspected by finding a prolonged thrombin time, but a normal Reptilase® time. Heparin may be inactivated by adding heparinase, Hepzyme™ or protamine sulfate to the sample. A repeat APTT will be normal if heparin was the culprit. In the absence of heparin, a prolonged APTT with a normal PT indicates either hemophilia or a circulating anticoagulant. A mixing test will exclude circulating anticoagulant. This involves mixing equal volumes of the patient's plasma with normal plasma and determining the APTT again. If the prolonged APTT is due to a clotting factor deficiency, the APTT should be corrected by the normal plasma to within 4 seconds of a simultaneously run control of normal plasma and buffer; otherwise a circulating anticoagulant should be suspected (see Chapter 13). Deficiencies of factors VIII, IX, and XI are associated with bleeding (see Chapters 6 and 7). Deficiencies of factors XII, prekallikrein and high MW kininogen are not associated with bleeding even though the APTT is prolonged.

A prolonged PT generally occurs with vitamin K deficiency, warfarin therapy or liver disease. Vitamin K deficiency occurs in individuals with extremely limited diets, such as those with biliary tract obstruction and those with malabsorption syndromes. Administration of vitamin K, 10 mg subcutaneously, will correct the PT within 24 hours if the abnormal clotting is due to deficiency of the vitamin. However, a prolonged PT in patients with hepatocellular liver disease will not be corrected. Patients with liver impairment have a complex coagulopathy, which includes both low levels of clotting factors and defects in platelet function and abnormal fibrinolysis (see Chapter 9). Lastly, a high hematocrit, as in polycythemia, artifactually prolongs the clotting times, because the decreased volume of plasma in such samples results in a relative excess of citrate in the sample collection tube.

If a specific abnormality is not identified by the platelet count, bleeding time, PFA-100, APTT or PT, patients with a history of bleeding should be referred to a coagulation consultant for further evaluation.

Intraoperative bleeding

Most surgical bleeding is due to local factors such as highly vascular tissues, anastomotic leaks, slipped ligatures or other technical problems, and poor wound healing. However, deficiencies or defects in circulating clotting factors may contribute. For example, oozing at the surgical site suggests impaired platelet function. This may be due to postoperative analgesics such as ketorolac, a NSAID, which inhibits platelet function. Very high intravenous doses of penicillin-type antibiotics, such as methicillin and carbenicillin, also impair platelet function. If packed red cells and plasma are given in large volumes, dilutional thrombocytopenia may occur, since these blood products lack platelets.

Another important cause of intraoperative bleeding is DIC (see Chapter 12). This may be triggered by prolonged hypotension, infection with organisms that produce endotoxin, or as a manifestation of a transfusion reaction. Characteristically, there is marked oozing from the wound as well as venepuncture sites. If there is a transfusion reaction, blood may appear in the urine. Laboratory studies will demonstrate a low platelet count, prolonged APTT and PT, and low fibrinogen levels. Treatment is directed towards any potential precipitating factor; for example, supporting blood pressure in patients with shock, giving antibiotics in those with sepsis and ensuring that the patient is receiving compatible blood. Platelets are infused, and the fibrinogen level raised by administering cryoprecipitate.

Postoperative bleeding

Bleeding in the postoperative period may be due to local factors or to a coagulopathy. When the coagulation screen and full blood count are normal, the most common causes of bleeding are local surgical factors (e.g. small bleeding vessel). Thrombocytopenia may occur because of dilution, platelet consumption or impaired platelet production. Patients with sepsis or adult respiratory distress syndrome are almost always thrombocytopenic; the platelet count rises when sepsis is controlled or lung function improves. Immune thrombocytopenias may be due to vancomycin or other antibiotics; intravenous famotidine appears to suppress platelet formation. Heparin-induced thrombocytopenia promotes platelet consumption and new thromboses; even heparin flushes of indwelling lines may trigger this syndrome (see Chapter 13).

Patients with mild-to-moderate hemophilia may not have been diagnosed preoperatively and may experience significant hemorrhage following surgery. Laboratory tests may reveal a prolonged APTT, but a normal PT, and deficiencies of factor VIII, factor IX or factor XI may be documented (though the APTT may be normal and measurement of the specific factor levels will be necessary to make the diagnosis). Giving the appropriate replacement therapy will control bleeding. Rarely, a patient will develop a circulating anticoagulant in the postoperative period (see Chapter 13). Factor VIII autoantibodies and antibodies to bovine proteins that cross-react with human factor V are both associated with bleeding. Factor VIII autoantibodies are readily recognized by a prolonged APTT test that fails to correct with normal plasma. Treatment with agents that bypass factor VIII in the clotting scheme, such as recombinant human factor VIIa or activated prothrombin complex concentrates, may provide hemostasis. Antibodies to factor V develop when fibrin glue, prepared with bovine thrombin, is sprayed onto serosal surfaces to control bleeding. After 1–2 weeks, the APTT and PT are found to be abnormal, and the factor V level decreased. The factor V antibodies may persist for weeks to months. If this is a cause of bleeding, recombinant human factor VIIa may secure hemostasis.

Bleeding associated with cardiopulmonary bypass surgery

Surgical trauma to vessels and tissues, as well as exposure of blood to artificial surfaces, induces activation of platelets, clotting factors and the fibrinolytic system. In addition, the continuous infusion of heparin during the procedure affects many aspects of coagulation. Thus, bleeding in patients undergoing cardiopulmonary bypass surgery is usually multifactorial. Platelet dysfunction, thrombocytopenia, and increased levels of tPA, thrombin–antithrombin complexes, plasmin-α_2–antiplasmin complexes and cross-linked FDPs characterize the coagulopathy.

Bleeding sufficiently severe to require re-exploration occurs in up to 7% of patients. The principal causes of bleeding in patients undergoing cardiopulmonary bypass surgery are:

- local surgical or anatomic factors
- preoperative medication affecting platelet function (e.g. aspirin, clopidogrel)
- hyperfibrinolysis
- inadequate postoperative neutralization of heparin with protamine.

In patients who were taking aspirin or clopidogrel preoperatively, administering desmopressin, 0.3 μg/kg in 50 mL of saline intravenously over 20 minutes, will often improve hemostasis. Transfusion of platelets may also be necessary. Bleeding due to excessive fibrinolysis generally occurs in patients undergoing more complicated procedures or repeat operations, and prolonged pump times. Aprotinin, a potent inhibitor of plasmin, is very effective in reducing bleeding in such patients. Aprotinin, at a dose of 2 million kallikrein inactivator units given as an intravenous bolus, added to the pump prime, and infused continuously during the procedure, provides a dry surgical field and reduces overall blood loss. However, aprotinin-induced inhibition of coagulation proteases may augment the prolongation of the activated clotting time by heparin, resulting in heparin underdosage. To avoid intraoperative thromboses due to inadequate heparin dosing, a method of heparin assessment insensitive to aprotinin must be used (e.g. the anti-Xa assay).

Massive, uncontrollable bleeding

Occasionally, patients undergoing surgery for repair of major trauma will have massive bleeding. The causes of such bleeding are multiple and include severe tissue injury releasing procoagulant tissue factor, intravascular coagulation with consumption of platelets and clotting factors, dilutional thrombocytopenia and excessive fibrinolysis. Attempts should be made to correct identifiable abnormalities; for example, administering platelets to raise a depressed platelet count, cryoprecipitate to improve the fibrinogen level, and infusing fresh frozen plasma if the APTT and PT are both prolonged. If bleeding persists, and especially if hemorrhage is life-threatening, recombinant human factor VIIa may be life-saving. There are anecdotal reports that this agent has lead to prompt cessation of spontaneous bleeding or hemorrhage following trauma or surgery, particularly if the coagulation screen is normal.

Key points – perioperative bleeding

- A carefully taken history is the best screening test for a coagulation disorder.
- If a bleeding tendency is suspected, the bleeding time or platelet function analyzer-100 test, the activated partial thromboplastin time and the prothrombin time may identify the cause.
- The management of surgical bleeding includes meticulous local hemostatic measures, as well as replacement of red cells, platelets and clotting factors.
- Consider vitamin K therapy in every postoperative patient with a prolonged prothrombin time.
- Recombinant human factor VIIa may be beneficial in the control of massive bleeding refractory to plasma, cryoprecipitate and platelet therapy.

Key references

Green D, Sanders J, Eiken M et al. Recombinant aprotinin in coronary artery bypass graft operations. *J Thorac Cardiovasc Surg* 1995; 110:963–70.

Kenet G, Walden R, Eldad A, Martinowitz U. Treatment of traumatic bleeding with recombinant factor VIIa. *Lancet* 1999;354:1879.

Kitchens CS. Surgery and Hemostasis. In: Kitchens CS, Alving BM, Kessler CM, eds. *Consultative Hemostasis and Thrombosis.* Philadelphia: WB Saunders, 2002: 463–80.

Martinowitz U, Kenet G, Segal E et al. Recombinant activated factor VII for adjunctive hemorrhage control in trauma. *J Trauma* 2001; 51:431–8.

Segal H, Hunt BJ. Aprotinin: pharmacological reduction of perioperative bleeding. *Lancet* 2000;355:1289–90.

12

Disseminated intravascular coagulation

DIC is an acquired syndrome characterized by intravascular activation of coagulation and deposition of fibrin within the microvasculature. This leads to organ ischemia and infarction. In acute DIC, the consumption of clotting factors and platelets in the diffusely distributed thrombi may lead to a hemorrhagic diathesis and clinical bleeding. The paradoxical combination of bleeding and thrombosis in a hypotensive patient with sepsis, cancer or obstetrical accident should raise suspicion of the syndrome, which is confirmed by examination of the blood film and coagulation studies. Some causes of DIC are listed in Table 12.1.

TABLE 12.1

Causes of disseminated intravascular coagulation

Infections

- Gram-negative or Gram-positive septicemia (endotoxin)
- Viruses (e.g. Epstein-Barr virus, cytomegalovirus, human immunodeficiency virus)
- Miliary tuberculosis
- Fungi
- Parasites (malaria, *Toxoplasma* spp.)

Release of tissue factor

- Malignancy, especially if disseminated
- Obstetric accident
- Preeclampsia
- Placental abruption
- Amniotic fluid embolism
- Extensive trauma, burns, surgery
- Aortic aneurysm
- Transfusion reaction

Clinical presentation

Acute DIC occurs with endotoxemia, extensive tissue trauma and, in women whose pregnancies are complicated by preeclampsia, placental abruption or amniotic fluid embolism. Acute DIC may also appear in patients experiencing hypotension or shock for any reason; for example, during a difficult surgical procedure or during a massive stroke or heart attack.

Chronic DIC is associated with malignancies, aortic aneurysms and large hemangiomas, and also is observed in women with a retained dead fetus. In patients with malignancies, the main risk factors are older age, male sex, advanced cancer and necrosis in the tumor. Most patients have adenocarcinomas of the lung, breast, prostate or colorectum. The survival of these patients is worse than that of cancer patients without DIC.

Pathophysiology

A common etiologic predisposing condition for the many disorders that induce DIC is excessive expression of TF. This transmembrane protein is expressed on the surface of monocytes and macrophages in patients with sepsis. In addition, increased levels of proinflammatory cytokines (e.g. IL-1 and TNFα), which are also synthesized by activated monocytes, are present in all situations associated with DIC. Following severe tissue trauma, particularly head injury, TF is liberated into the circulation. It is also released as a result of intravascular hemolysis, as occurs during transfusion reactions or attacks of *Plasmodium falciparum* malaria. In patients with placental abruption, increased intrauterine pressure may force TF-rich decidual fragments into the maternal circulation and, in women with amniotic fluid embolism, fluids and tissues containing TF enter the maternal circulation.

The consequence of this extensive exposure to TF is a profound activation of coagulation and the generation of large amounts of thrombin. Thrombin promotes platelet activation and aggregates form, which occlude the microvasculature and result in thrombocytopenia. Thrombin becomes bound to antithrombin and thrombomodulin, and these proteins are soon consumed. Following binding to thrombomodulin, thrombin activates the anticoagulant protein C, which also becomes depleted, predisposing to microvascular thrombosis. As part of the acute inflammatory reaction, raised levels of the C4B-binding protein result in the binding of more free protein S, and therefore render it unavailable to be a cofactor of the anticoagulant protein C. PAI-1 is increased by the inflammatory reaction out of proportion to the levels of tPA, resulting in depressed fibrinolysis. Fibrin is formed, but its removal is impaired, leading to thrombosis of small and midsize vessels. The passage of erythrocytes through partially occluded vessels, and the macrophage activation that accompanies DIC, lead to red cell fragmentation and microangiopathic hemolytic anemia.

Diagnosis

The characteristic coagulation changes in acute and chronic DIC are summarized in Table 12.2.

TABLE 12.2

Characteristic findings in acute and chronic disseminated intravascular coagulation (DIC)

Observation	Acute DIC	Chronic DIC
Platelet count	Decreased	Decreased
APTT and PT	Prolonged	Variable
Fibrinogen	Decreased	Variable
Fibrin degradation products	Increased	Increased
Coagulation inhibitors*	Decreased	Decreased
Plasminogen	Decreased	Decreased
Tissue plasminogen activator	Increased	Decreased
Plasminogen activator-1	Increased	Increased
Anemia	Present	Present
Hemostasis	Persistent oozing	Thrombosis

*Inhibitors are antithrombin, proteins C, S and Z, and tissue factor pathway inhibitor. APPT, activated partial thromboplastin time; PT, prothrombin time.

In acute DIC, platelets, clotting factors (especially factors V and VIII) and fibrinogen are rapidly consumed. In addition, fibrin degradation products, such as fragments X and E, are generated. These bind to fibrin and enhance the activity of tPA, resulting in more rapid lysis of clots. Depletion of platelets and clotting factors, coupled with the increased fibrinolytic activity, results in persistent oozing from the gastrointestinal and genitourinary tracts, as well as from venepuncture and other sites of tissue invasion. There may also be signs of organ ischemia, because of micro- or macrovascular thrombosis.

In chronic DIC, the rate of enhanced production of some clotting factors is greater than their rate of consumption and this may result in elevated concentrations of fibrinogen and factor VIII. Platelet levels, however, usually remain low. The raised levels of fibrinogen and factor VIII and ongoing consumption of clotting factor inhibitors and components of the fibrinolytic system (plasminogen and tPA), shifts the hemostatic balance towards thrombosis.

Acute DIC should be considered in any patient with sepsis, shock, extensive tissue trauma or an obstetric accident that experiences bleeding. A platelet count, APTT, PT, and measurements of fibrinogen and FDPs are indicated. The DIC Subcommittee of the International Society on Thrombosis and Haematology has developed a scoring system primarily for research studies on overt DIC based on the above criteria, and a second scoring system for chronic DIC that includes measurements of antithrombin and protein C, as well as molecular markers of coagulation activation.

Treatment

The treatment of DIC is primarily directed towards the underlying cause, but more specific measures are summarized in Table 12.3.

Acute disseminated intravascular coagulation. Antibiotics should be given for sepsis, volume expanders for shock and oxygen for hypoxia; evacuation of the uterus should be performed for obstetric accidents. In addition, therapy is also directed to control abnormalities of hemostasis. Patients with acute DIC may have profound bleeding, usually because of hypofibrinogenemia. Fibrinogen levels may be

TABLE 12.3

Treatment of acute and chronic disseminated intravascular coagulation (DIC)

Treatment	Acute DIC	Chronic DIC
Address underlying cause	Yes	Yes
Cryoprecipitate	10 bags	No
Platelet transfusions	If platelet count < 20 × 10^9/L or bleeding present	No
Fresh frozen plasma	Infrequently indicated	No
Anticoagulants	Recombinant human activated protein C in non-bleeding septic patients	Heparin, LMWH

LMWH, low molecular weight heparin.

increased by administering cryoprecipitate. The amount of fibrinogen in each bag, prepared from 250 mL of plasma, is 300–400 mg, and giving ten bags should increase the fibrinogen level by 1 g/L, which should control most bleeding. Persistent oozing may be due to severe thrombocytopenia, as well as platelet dysfunction resulting from elevated levels of FDPs. Administering platelets should elevate the count and help stem bleeding. Prolongation of the APTT and PT, are usually caused by low fibrinogen concentrations and decreased levels of factors V and VIII, is best corrected by administering cryoprecipitate, which is rich in fibrinogen and factor VIII. Platelet transfusions may also provide factor V, which is present in the intracellular granules.

Because DIC results from activation of coagulation, there has been considerable interest in examining whether anticoagulants might be beneficial. Initial experience with heparin in patients with acute DIC was disastrous; bleeding was accentuated and mortality increased. However, more physiological approaches have recently been investigated.

Recombinant human activated protein C (raPC) was studied in a large trial of septic patients with evidence of multiple organ dysfunction; raPC, 24 µg/kg/hour for 96 hours, decreased mortality from 30.8% to 24.7% (p = 0.005). Serious bleeding was only modestly increased, from 2.0% to 3.5% (p = 0.06).

Antithrombin concentrate has also been studied in septic patients with DIC. A meta-analysis of six small trials showed a reduction of mortality from 47% to 32%. Bleeding rates were not reported.

Chronic DIC. The management of chronic DIC also begins with efforts to manage the underlying disorder; for example, encouraging uterine evacuation of a retained dead fetus. However, the most common cause of chronic DIC is cancer, and many of the tumors are resistant to therapy. Heparin is given to control some of the manifestations of DIC, such as migratory thrombophlebitis, venous thromboembolism and fibrin deposition in the lung. Previously, unfractionated heparin was given as a continuous intravenous infusion of 500 U/hour or as subcutaneous doses of 10 000 U up to every 8 hours. More recently, subcutaneously administered LMWHs have proven safe and effective. The dose should be titrated against the clinical response and laboratory measurement of the fibrinogen level and platelet count.

Key points – disseminated intravascular coagulation

- Persistent oozing from venepuncture sites in a septic patient, or massive vaginal bleeding in an obstetric patient, suggests disseminated intravascular coagulation (DIC).
- Hypofibrinogenemia usually indicates acute DIC, but the fibrinogen level is often normal or elevated in chronic DIC and is not a reliable marker of the condition.
- Treatment is directed towards the underlying cause of the DIC; bleeding is controlled with cryoprecipitate and platelet infusions.

Key references

Bernard GR, Vincent JL, Laterre PF et al. Efficacy and safety of recombinant human activated protein C for severe sepsis. *N Engl J Med* 2001;344:699–709.

Levi M, ten Cate H. Disseminated intravascular coagulation. *N Engl J Med* 1999;341:586–92.

Levi M, de Jonge E, van der Poll T, ten Cate H. Disseminated intravascular coagulation. *Thromb Haemost* 1999;82:695–705.

Sallah S, Wan JY, Nguyen NP et al. Disseminated intravascular coagulation in solid tumors: clinical and pathologic study. *Thromb Haemost* 2001;86:828–33.

Taylor FB Jr, Toh CH, Hoots WK et al. Towards definition, clinical and laboratory criteria, and a scoring system for disseminated intravascular coagulation. *Thromb Haemost* 2001; 86:1327–30.

Toh CH, Dennis M. Disseminated intravascular coagulation: old disease, new hope. *BMJ* 2003:327: 974–7.

Warren BL, Eid, A, Singer P et al. High dose antithrombin III in severe sepsis: a randomized controlled trial. *JAMA* 2001;286:1869–78.

A bleeding state may arise either because the patient develops a spontaneous pathological anticoagulant (often an antibody against one of the clotting factors) or, much more commonly, from therapy with an anticoagulant or antithrombotic drug.

Pathological anticoagulants

There are two main types of pathological anticoagulants (which are so-named because they prolong clotting times in vitro): those directed against a specific clotting factor; and those directed against phospholipid-binding proteins. The former are associated with bleeding and the latter with thrombosis (see page 111). Almost all of these anticoagulants are antibodies, and most are considered to be autoimmune in origin.

Antibodies to specific clotting factors (acquired hemophilia). The most common spontaneously arising anticoagulant is an autoantibody directed against factor VIII, though it is, overall, a relatively rare condition.

Clinical presentation. Affected individuals are usually elderly and often have cancer or other autoimmune diseases (e.g. asthma or rheumatoid arthritis), but 50% have no other disease apparent when the inhibitor is first detected. Rarely, these antibodies appear during, or after, an otherwise normal pregnancy. They come to medical attention because of bleeding in the skin or muscles after relatively minor trauma, gastrointestinal or genitourinary bleeding, or occult blood loss that may lead to profound anemia.

Diagnosis. The diagnosis is suspected when an elderly person, who has tolerated previous surgery and trauma without bleeding, has unexplained hemorrhage. The APTT is prolonged, but the prothrombin time is normal, which suggests reduced activity of clotting factors VIII, IX or XI. Specific assay shows a reduced level of factor VIII; mixing and incubating the patient's plasma with normal plasma fails to correct the APTT or the factor VIII level. A quantitative assay, the Bethesda method, indicates the titer (potency) of the anticoagulant.

Treatment is directed towards control of bleeding and suppression of the antibody (Table 13.1). It is important to measure the titer of the inhibitor against both porcine and human factor VIII. If the antihuman activity is above 5 Bethesda U/mL, or the antiporcine above 10, neither human nor porcine factor VIII is likely to be effective in arresting hemorrhage, and recombinant human factor VIIa or activated prothrombin complex concentrate may be appropriate.

Patients with factor VIII autoantibodies should be given prednisone, 1 mg/kg/day, immediately, because in about one-third of patients the anticoagulant will disappear within 6 weeks with this therapy. Occasionally, intravenous IgG, 1 g/kg daily for 2 days, will lead to a dramatic disappearance of the inhibitor, though the effect is usually transient. Patients with inhibitors resistant to corticosteroids and IgG require immunosuppression with cyclophosphamide, ciclosporin, rituximab or similar agents.

TABLE 13.1

Comparison of products for the management of bleeding in patients with factor VIII inhibitors (autoantibodies)

Product	Effectiveness	Allergy	Thrombo-cytopenia	Thrombosis
Porcine VIII	Initially 80%; but resistance may occur with continued use owing to a rise in antibody level	5–10%	5–10%	No
Recombinant human factor VIIa	94%	1–2%	Infrequent	Reported
Activated prothrombin complex concentrate	80%	5–10%	Infrequent	Reported

Anticoagulant antibodies arising in association with other diseases.
Inhibitors directed against a variety of clotting factors may appear
during the course of malignant disease, such as myeloma,
macroglobulinemia, lymphoma and other cancers (Table 13.2).

The inhibitors are either antibodies or paraproteins that inhibit the
function of one or more hemostatic proteins. For example, myeloma
proteins may alter the ability of fibrinogen monomers to polymerize,
or factor XIII to cross-link nascent fibrin strands. Immunoglobulins
may inhibit vWF multimerization, altering its ability to support platelet
adhesion or aggregation. Amyloid proteins may absorb factor X,
leading to a bleeding diathesis. Treatment is directed against the
underlying disease, but some of these paraproteins may be removed
by plasmapheresis or suppressed by chemotherapy. Bleeding may be
brought under control by the administration of the inhibited clotting
factor or by use of recombinant human factor VIIa.

Antiphospholipid antibodies (i.e. lupus anticoagulant and
anticardiolipin antibody) are autoantibodies that inhibit various
natural or artificial phospholipid–protein complexes. Such complexes

TABLE 13.2

**Pathological inhibitors of hemostasis associated with
lymphoproliferative diseases**

Disease	Clotting factor	Mechanism	Treatment
Myeloma	Fibrinogen	Poor polymerization, gelatinous clots	Chemotherapy, transplantation
Macro-globulinemia	von Willebrand factor	Absorption of multimers	Plasmapheresis
Amyloidosis	Factor X	Absorption of factor X	Splenectomy
Lymphomas and other cancers	Any factor	Autoantibodies to clotting factor	Immuno-suppression, chemotherapy

form when phospholipids, especially phosphatidylserine, are exposed on cell membranes. These phospholipids are immediately complexed by proteins such as β_2-glycoprotein-1, annexins, prothrombin and other clotting factors. Antibodies produced against these complexes may alter the tissue bearing the phospholipid–protein complex; for example, damage to platelets results in thrombocytopenia, to nerve tissue produces cerebral dysfunction, to the placenta causes intrauterine fetal death, and to endothelial cells leads to thrombosis. A variety of tests are used that detect either the ability of the antibody to inhibit the clotting mechanism, in the case of lupus anticoagulant, or to bind to phospholipids, such as cardiolipin or synthetic hexagonal phase phospholipids, in the case of anticardiolipin antibody. The 'lupus anticoagulant' is an autoantibody detected by its ability to prolong the APTT test. While it is important to note that these antibodies may appear to be anticoagulants in vitro, they are associated with thrombosis in vivo.

Diagnosis and management. The lupus anticoagulant is detected by tests using low concentrations of phospholipids, such as the dilute Russell viper venom time or the dilute tissue thromboplastin time. Anticardiolipin antibodies are detected by an enzyme-linked immunosorbent assay specific for IgG or IgM anticardiolipin antibodies.

The antibodies are associated with arterial and venous thrombosis, neuropsychiatric disorders, recurrent miscarriages, heart valve thrombi and livedo reticularis (thrombi in skin vessels). The recurrence rate for thrombosis is high, often necessitating long-term antithrombotic therapy. Secondary antiphospholipid antibodies are also detected in patients with various types of malignancy, infections such as syphilis and HIV, and the use of certain drugs. However, the incidence of thrombosis is much lower than in individuals with primary antiphospholipid antibodies.

Rarely, patients with systemic lupus erythematosus develop antibodies directed against specific clotting factors, such as factor VIII or prothrombin. Under these circumstances, hemorrhage rather than thrombosis is the major clinical manifestation.

Therapeutic anticoagulants and antithrombotic agents

Five major classes of antithrombotic agents are in clinical use:

- agents inhibiting platelet function (aspirin, thienopyridines, Gp IIb/IIIa inhibitors)
- heparins (unfractionated heparin, LMWH, pentasaccharide)
- coumarin derivatives (warfarin, acenocoumarol)
- direct thrombin inhibitors (argatroban, bivalirudin, lepirudin, ximelagatran)
- thrombolytic agents (streptokinase, urokinase, tPA).

Before starting any antithrombotic therapy, it is essential to consider the balance between reducing the chances of thromboembolism and increasing the risk of bleeding in each individual patient. Furthermore, antithrombotic therapy should be reviewed regularly to ensure that the hemorrhagic potential of the patient has not changed (e.g. the development of renal or hepatic failure) and that the current dose of drugs is appropriate.

Bleeding associated with antithrombotic agents may be major, defined as:

- a decline in the hemoglobin of more than 20 g/L
- the need for transfusion of 2 or more units of blood
- intracranial, retroperitoneal or fatal bleeding.

Minor bleeding includes all other bleeding, such as skin bruising, wound hematoma, epistaxis and hematuria. (In some clinical studies, a bleeding index has been used to define major bleeding. It is calculated as the number of units of blood transfused plus the difference between the prebleeding and postbleeding hemoglobin levels in g/dL, where a value of 2 or more indicates major bleeding.)

Inhibitors of platelet function. Some characteristics of platelet function inhibitors are shown in Table 13.3.

Aspirin and other NSAIDs alter platelet function by inhibiting both cyclooxygenase-1 and -2. This results in impaired generation of thromboxane A_2 and prostacyclin. Because thromboxane is a major inducer of platelet aggregation and vasoconstriction, treatment with aspirin and NSAIDs inhibits platelet function. A meta-analysis of 287 studies involving 135 000 patients showed that antiplatelet therapy

TABLE 13.3

Some characteristics of platelet function inhibitors

Characteristic	Aspirin and NSAIDs	Thienopyridines	Glycoprotein IIb/IIIa inhibitors
Route of administration	Oral	Oral	Intravenous
Site of action	Cyclooxygenase enzymes	Adenosine diphosphate receptor	Membrane glycoprotein
Duration of action	1–7 days	Up to 2 weeks	≥ 4–12 hours

NSAIDs, non-steroidal anti-inflammatory drugs.

reduced the risk of having a recurrence of heart attack, stroke or peripheral arterial occlusion by at least 25%. The risk of major bleeding with antiplatelet drugs is increased by about 50% (odds ratio 1.6), which represents about one or two additional major extracranial bleeds per 1000 patient-years. The regular use of aspirin is associated with a twofold increase in the risk of upper gastrointestinal bleeding. In five large clinical trials comparing aspirin with placebo, upper gastrointestinal bleeding increased from 1.1 (placebo) to 2.5 (aspirin) major bleeds per 1000 patient-years, and the frequency of all bleeds was doubled. Therapy with other NSAIDs is also complicated by bleeding; some provoke more bleeding than others. For example, the risk with ibuprofen is 2.9, indomethacin 6.3 and piroxicam 18.0. This risk may be modified by the concomitant use of proton pump inhibitors.

Aspirin irreversibly acetylates platelet cyclooxygenase; the impairment lasts for the life of the platelet exposed to aspirin. Since the platelet life span is approximately 10 days, a week with no aspirin exposure is required before most of the platelets are fully functional. NSAIDs are reversible inhibitors of cyclooxygenase, so their inhibitory effect on platelet function is only transitory, lasting about 24 hours. However, they alter the mucosal barrier of the gastric lining, and this plays a major role in their propensity to cause gastrointestinal bleeding.

Thienopyridine derivatives (ticlopidine and clopidogrel) inhibit the binding of ADP to its platelet receptor P2Y12. The onset of action is gradual; maximal inhibition takes up to 1 week to achieve and the effect persists for up to 2 weeks after the agents are discontinued. Because clopidogrel is more potent than ticlopidine, and has been much less frequently associated with agranulocytosis and thrombotic thrombocytopenic purpura, it has replaced ticlopidine in clinical practice. The risks of major bleeding with clopidogrel are low, and no higher than with aspirin; however, major bleeding may occur with surgery. The combination of clopidogrel and aspirin is associated with more bleeding than with aspirin alone; 3.7% versus 2.7% in one major trial. Most bleeding has been from the gastrointestinal tract and at sites of arterial puncture.

Inhibitors of platelet Gp IIb/IIIa impair the binding of fibrinogen to its platelet receptor, thereby preventing platelet aggregation. Most are used in the management of coronary heart disease and are given intravenously. Abciximab is a humanized mouse monoclonal antibody, and eptifibatide and tirofiban are small molecule inhibitors of the platelet fibrinogen receptor. The duration of inhibition of platelet function (i.e. > 50% inhibition) is much longer with abciximab (12 hours) than with eptifibatide or tirofiban (4 hours). The incidence of major bleeding with these agents has been about 0.1% in several large clinical trials, which is not significantly different from placebo. Severe thrombocytopenia is a very serious adverse effect with an incidence of 0.1–0.5%. However, despite platelet counts as low as 1×10^9/L, bleeding has been minimal and most patients have been managed with platelet infusions.

Treatment of bleeding due to platelet inhibiting agents. Bleeding due to aspirin and NSAIDs is usually from the gastrointestinal tract and often responds to withdrawal of the drug and treatment with proton pump inhibitors. Occasionally, intravenous desmopressin, 0.3 µg/kg, will help to control bleeding from various sites, such as the nose, gastrointestinal and genitourinary tracts. Bleeding due to longer acting agents, such as the thienopyridines, may require platelet transfusions. For major or life-threatening bleeding associated with Gp IIb/IIIa inhibitors, platelets or recombinant human factor VIIa may be effective.

Heparins. Three classes of heparins are in current clinical use (Table 13.4):

- unfractionated heparin
- LMWH
- pentasaccharide (fondaparinux).

While the principal mode of action is by activation of antithrombin, each agent has unique effects on coagulation. Unfractionated heparin has the shortest half-life, LMWHs have half-lives of 3–4 hours depending on the specific product, and fondaparinux has the longest half-life (17 hours). The ratio of antifactor Xa activity to antithrombin activity is 1.0 for unfractionated heparin and 2–4 for LMWHs; fondaparinux has no antithrombin activity. Although the antithrombin activity of LMWH and fondaparinux is weak or non-existent, their ability to inhibit factor Xa, and in the case of LMWH, to release TFPI, provides powerful antithrombotic activity.

Bleeding risk. The principal adverse effect of heparin is bleeding. In patients treated with full-dose intravenous unfractionated heparin, the rate of major bleeding ranges from 0% to 7%, and fatal bleeding from 0% to 2%. For LMWH, the rate of major bleeding is 0% to 3% and of fatal bleeding from 0% to 0.8%. In several trials in which heparin and LMWH were compared directly, significantly less bleeding

TABLE 13.4

Properties of unfractionated heparin, low molecular weight heparin (LMWH) and pentasaccharide

Property	Heparin	LMWH	Pentasaccharide
Bind antithrombin	Yes	Yes	Yes
Inhibit thrombin	Yes	Weak	No
Inhibit factor Xa	Yes	Yes	Yes
Inactivate platelet-bound factor Xa	No	Yes	Yes
Release tissue factor pathway inhibitor	Yes	Yes	No
Half-life	90 minutes	3–4 hours	13–21 hours

occurred with LMWH. The factors that predispose to bleeding include older age, renal failure and concomitant aspirin therapy. The sites of bleeding are diverse and can be gastrointestinal, genitourinary, intrapulmonary, retroperitoneal or intracranial.

Bleeds into the epidural space, resulting in spinal cord compression, are particularly dangerous, and have been reported when epidural catheters, used for analgesia, are placed or removed within a short time of an injection of anticoagulant. Additional factors predisposing to epidural hematomas are older age, female sex, and concomitant use of aspirin, ketorolac (an NSAID) or warfarin.

The bleeding risk with fondaparinux, 2.5 mg/day, after surgery has been compared with LMWH (enoxaparin) and the pooled estimates from four trials (3616 patients) were 2.7% and 1.7%, respectively. Thus, there is a small increase in the risk of hemorrhage with fondaparinux compared with LMWH.

Treatment. The management of bleeding due to heparins begins with immediate discontinuation of the agent. Since unfractionated heparin has a relatively short half-life (about 90 minutes), the administration of an antidote is rarely required. However, if bleeding is brisk or life-threatening, protamine sulfate may be given intravenously at a dose of 1 mg for each 100 units of heparin suspected to be in the circulation; in practice, because of a delay of at least 2–3 hours in obtaining the drug in most institutions, half the calculated dose may be given. A large dose of protamine may produce hypotension, bleeding and severe allergic reactions in certain individuals. Protamine sulfate only neutralizes the antithrombin activity of LMWH rather than its antifactor Xa activity and does not affect fondaparinux; it may, therefore, be an ineffective antidote for these drugs. The use of recombinant human factor VIIa should be considered in patients with life-threatening bleeding due to LMWH or fondaparinux until more specific antagonists become available.

Heparin-induced thrombocytopenia is a serious complication, because it is associated with the development of arterial and venous thrombosis. It occurs in up to 3% of patients treated with unfractionated heparin and in fewer than 1% receiving LMWH, and has not been reported with fondaparinux. It usually occurs after 5 days of heparin treatment, or earlier if there has been previous heparin exposure. Platelet counts generally decline by 50% or more, but bleeding is rarely encountered; rather there may be life- and limb-threatening thrombosis. All heparin must be promptly discontinued; this includes heparin flushes and heparin-coated catheters. Furthermore, HIT results in activation of coagulation, so that the risk of new thromboses continues for weeks after exposure to heparin. The use of a non-heparin anticoagulant, such as the direct thrombin inhibitors hirudin or argatroban, should be considered in all patients and, when the platelet count has recovered, an oral anticoagulant may be started, but at a lower than normal initial dose to prevent a sudden lowering of the anticoagulant protein C level.

Vitamin K cycle

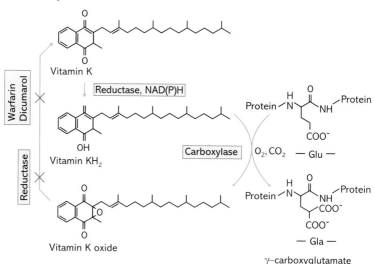

Figure 13.1 Mode of action of coumarin. Vitamin K absorbed from the gut is reduced to vitamin KH_2, and serves as the coenzyme for the carboxylase that completes the synthesis of clotting factors II, VII, IX and X, as well as proteins C, S and Z. Vitamin KH_2 becomes oxidized and requires the action of a reductase to cycle it back to its original form. Warfarin inhibits this reductase and thereby interferes with the vitamin K cycle. (Adapted from Dowd P et al. *Science* 1995;269:1684.) Glu, glutamine; Gla, glutamic acid.

Coumarins (e.g. warfarin) are orally active antithrombotic agents that inhibit the enzymatic reduction of vitamin K (Figure 13.1). This prevents the carboxylation of factors II, VII, IX and X, which is essential for their participation in the coagulation system. This effect on coagulation may be monitored by measuring the PT, which is sensitive to the activity levels of clotting factors II, VII and X. The international normalized ratio (INR) refers to the standardization of the PT in general use for monitoring warfarin. The target INR for different indications is given in Table 13.5.

The most important adverse effect of coumarins is bleeding. In most individuals, it takes 3–5 days after exposure to warfarin for clotting factor levels decline to the extent that thrombosis is prevented or that

TABLE 13.5

Target internal normalized ratio (INR) for different indications

Indication	Target INR
Pulmonary embolus	2.5
Proximal deep vein thrombosis	2.5
Calf vein thrombus	2.5
Recurrence of venous thromboembolism when no longer on warfarin therapy	2.5
Recurrence of venous thromboembolism whilst on warfarin therapy	3.5*
Symptomatic inherited thrombophilia	2.5
Antiphospholipid syndrome	2.5
Non-rheumatic atrial fibrillation	2.5
Atrial fibrillation due to rheumatic heart disease, congenital heart disease or thyrotoxicosis	2.5
Cardioversion	2.5
Mural thrombus	2.5
Cardiomyopathy	2.5
Mechanical prosthetic heart valve	3.5

*Consider switching to heparin.
Data from *Br J Haematol* 1998;101:374–87.

bleeding is a risk. The risk of bleeding rises with the increasing INR, and it rises more sharply when the INR exceeds 3.0.

Bleeding risk. The risk of bleeding with coumarins is strongly related to the patient's vitamin K status. Patients on diets with a restricted vitamin K content, or those unable to eat because of recent surgery, neurological disease or other disorders, are very sensitive to even small doses of coumarins. In addition, those unable to absorb vitamin K because of diarrhea, biliary tract obstruction or malabsorption syndromes are at very high risk of bleeding, and coumarins should be administered cautiously. An index to assess the risk of bleeding in hospitalized patients starting anticoagulants has been developed by Landefeld. Factors associated with an increased risk for bleeding were the number of specific comorbid conditions (e.g. serious cardiac disease, liver dysfunction, renal insufficiency and poor general status), heparin use in patients over the age of 60, exceeding the therapeutic range (PT more than two times control) and worsening liver function.

Drug interactions. Many drugs affect the response to coumarins; some examples are listed in Table 13.6. These drugs enhance the effect of coumarins in a variety of ways.

- They inhibit the hepatic microsomal enzyme systems, cytochromes P450, that metabolize coumarins.
- They displace coumarin from its protein binding sites, increasing the amount of free drug.
- They alter the synthesis of clotting factors by interfering with the regeneration of reduced vitamin K or by other mechanisms.

Increases in the INR have been reported with a variety of herbal preparations, such as garlic, ginkgo, danshen, dong quai and papaya. Garlic and ginkgo inhibit platelet function, danshen decreases the clearance of coumarins and dong quai contains coumarins. Bleeding is also more common in individuals with certain polymorphisms in the cytochrome P450 enzyme (CYP2C9), which alter the metabolism of coumarins. These patients require smaller drug doses and tend to have INRs that exceed the therapeutic range. In the future, they may be identified prospectively by genetic studies and either treated with smaller doses of coumarins or given alternative anticoagulants. The

TABLE 13.6

Drugs potentiating the effect of coumarins

Antibiotics

- Azoles (co-trimoxazole, fluconazole, metronidazole, miconazole)
- Cephalosporins
- Macrolides (erythromycin, azithromycin)
- Quinolones (ciprofloxacin)
- Isoniazid

Cardiac drugs

- Amiodarone
- Clofibrate
- Propafenone
- Propranolol
- Sulfinpyrazone

Antipyretics and anti-inflammatory drugs

- Acetaminophen (paracetamol)
- Non-steroidal anti-inflammatory drugs (diclofenac sodium, piroxicam)

Histamine H_2-blockers

- Cimetidine
- Omeprazole

Herbal medicines

- Garlic
- Ginkgo
- Danshen
- Dong quai
- Papaya

Other drugs

- Statins (e.g. simvastatin)
- Sertraline
- Tamoxifen
- Thyroid hormone
- Ticlopidine
- Vitamin E

ingestion of a small amount of alcohol stimulates the P450 enzymes and increases the metabolism of coumarins, but larger quantities enhance the anticoagulant effects and promote bleeding. The greatest risk for hemorrhage with coumarins occurs in the first month of therapy, and the risk of life-threatening bleeding is 0.5–1% per year thereafter.

Treatment of bleeding due to coumarin begins with cessation of the anticoagulant. It is always important to consider the possibility of an underlying structural lesion (e.g. an ulcer or neoplasm), particularly if bleeding occurs while the INR is in the therapeutic range. Guidance on further therapeutic interventions depends on the INR and the severity of bleeding (Table 13.7).

Direct thrombin inhibitors. Several direct thrombin inhibitors are currently available or in clinical trials and include lepirudin, bivalirudin and argatroban. Lepirudin and bivalirudin inhibit both the exosite and catalytic site of thrombin, while argatroban inhibits only the catalytic site. The drugs are given intravenously and have a half-life of 25–50 minutes. Lepirudin and bivalirudin are metabolized by the kidney, and argatroban by the liver. Major dose modification is

TABLE 13.7

Recommendations for management of bleeding and excessive anticoagulation

INR and severity of bleeding	Intervention
3.0 < INR < 6.0 (target INR 2.5) No bleeding or minor bleeding	1. Reduce or stop warfarin dose 2. Restart warfarin when INR < 5.0
6.0 < INR < 8.0 No bleeding or minor bleeding	1. Stop warfarin 2. Restart when INR < 5.0
INR > 8.0 No bleeding or minor bleeding	1. Stop warfarin 2. Restart warfarin when INR < 5.0 3. If other risk factors for bleeding present, give vitamin K, 0.5–2.5 mg orally
Major bleeding	1. Stop warfarin 2. Give prothrombin complex concentrate, 50 U/kg or fresh frozen plasma 15 mL/kg 3. Give vitamin K, 5 mg orally or i.v.

INR, international normalized ratio.
From *Br J Haematol* 1998;101:374–87.

required if lepirudin or bivalirudin is given to patients with renal failure, or argatroban to those with liver impairment.

Bivalirudin is given intravenously in doses based on body weight. In the HERO-2 trial, the APTT was monitored 12 and 24 hours after treatment was initiated; times exceeding 150 seconds were associated with more frequent bleeding. Patients receiving lepirudin and argatroban must be closely monitored. With lepirudin, the APTT is measured 4 hours after the initial dose and repeated daily; it should not exceed 2.5 times the control. With argatroban, the APTT is measured 2 hours after the dose and should not exceed three times the control. Values of APTT above 100 seconds are regularly associated with hemorrhage, which may be severe.

Ximelagatran is rapidly absorbed following oral administration and is converted to melagatran, a potent thrombin inhibitor. It binds competitively to the active site of clot-bound, as well as free, thrombin thus preventing the further conversion of fibrinogen to fibrin. Clinical trials have assessed its efficacy in prevention of stroke in atrial fibrillation, prevention and treatment of venous thromboembolism, and prevention of thromboembolic events after myocardial infarction. Ximelagatran is in the preregistration phase of development and is not yet licensed.

Treatment. There are no specific antidotes for direct thrombin inhibitors; however, their relatively short half-lives usually limit the duration of bleeding. If necessary, hemodialysis may help to clear the agent.

Thrombolytic agents. The process of thrombus dissolution begins with the binding of circulating plasminogen and plasminogen activators to the fibrin clot. The plasminogen is converted to plasmin and plasmin digests fibrin. Plasmin that escapes from the clot is neutralized by circulating antiplasmin. When pharmacological doses of thrombolytic agents (e.g. streptokinase and tPA) are administered, plasmin formation within the circulation is greatly enhanced and it digests circulating fibrinogen as well as the fibrin in the thrombus. Fibrinogenolysis promotes bleeding not only locally, particularly at catheter and operation sites, but also systemically, because it reduces

the concentration of circulating fibrinogen. Three thrombolytic agents
are in current use:

- streptokinase
- urokinase
- tPA.

Streptokinase and urokinase activate both free and fibrin-bound
plasminogen, while tPA mainly activates fibrin-bound plasminogen.
Unfortunately, the expectation that tPA would be associated with less
bleeding has not been borne out by clinical practice. A meta-analysis
performed by Sasahara et al. demonstrated bleeding complications in
29% of patients receiving streptokinase, 15% receiving tPA and
10% receiving urokinase. In another study of patients with myocardial
infarction treated with tPA, the incidence of intracranial bleeding was
0.95%; 53% died during hospitalization and another 25% had residual
neurological deficits. A study that compared tPA with streptokinase
showed more strokes in the tPA group (1.33% versus 0.94%). The
major risk factors for bleeding are older age, systolic blood pressure
above 140 mmHg and history of stroke. Any interruption of vascular
integrity may lead to hemorrhage; for example, placement of a femoral
sheath for catheter insertion or a venepuncture to obtain blood
samples. Spontaneous bleeding from the gastrointestinal tract or into
the retroperitoneum also occurs, but the main concern is the
unpredictability of intracranial bleeding.

Treatment. Patients receiving thrombolytic agents should be under
continuous observation, usually in an intensive care unit. Invasive
procedures should be avoided if at all possible but, if necessary,
pressure should be applied to sites used for needle or catheter
placement. Patients should be warned to avoid activities that may
lead to bleeding, such as heavy coughing, straining at stool or walking
without assistance. If major bleeding occurs during the infusion of a
thrombolytic agent, the drug should be stopped immediately, and a full
blood count and coagulation screen performed. These agents disappear
from the circulation within minutes and often nothing more needs to
be done. However, if bleeding is profuse or in a vulnerable area, an
antifibrinolytic agent may be infused intravenously. Either EACA, 5 g
given slowly over 20 minutes followed by a continuous infusion of

1 g/hour, or tranexamic acid, 0.5–1.0 g every 8 hours, would be appropriate. If thrombocytopenia or reduced fibrinogen levels are present, platelets or fresh frozen plasma may be helpful. Once there has been exposure to these drugs, thrombi may be more resistant to subsequent attempts at lysis.

Key points – anticoagulants and antithrombotic agents

Pathological anticoagulants
- A pathological anticoagulant should be suspected when major, unprovoked bleeding occurs in a previously well person.

Pharmacological anticoagulants
- Serious bleeding associated with aspirin and other non-steroidal anti-inflammatory agents may be controlled by platelet transfusion and, if minor but troublesome, with desmopressin.
- A decline in hemoglobin in a patient receiving heparin, LMWH or coumarin anticoagulant should prompt an exhaustive search for a source of bleeding.
- Coumarins should be used cautiously, if at all, in patients with poor oral intake.
- The direct thrombin inhibitors that are currently available require close monitoring using the activated partial thromboplastin time, and dose adjustments for liver disease (argatroban) or renal disease (lepirudin).

Thrombolytic agents
- Thrombolytic agents are associated with a risk of intracranial hemorrhage of nearly 1%; they should be administered in intensive care units and stopped immediately if signs of bleeding occur.

Key references

Aithal G, Day CP, Kesteven PJL, Daly AK. Association of polymorphisms in the cytochrome P450 CYP2C9 with warfarin dose requirement and risk of bleeding complications. *Lancet* 1998;353:717–19.

Alving BM, ed. *Blood Components and Pharmacologic Agents*. Bethesda: AABB Press, 2000:367.

Antithrombotic Trialists' Collaboration. Collaborative meta-analysis of randomised trials of antiplatelet therapy for prevention of death, myocardial infarction, and stroke in high risk patients. *BMJ* 2002;324:71–86.

Becker RC, Fintel DJ, Green D. *Antithrombotic Therapy*. 2nd edn. Caddo, Oklahoma: Professional Communications, 2002:301–21.

Berkowitz SD, Harrington RH, Rund MM, Tcheng JE. Acute profound thrombocytopenia after c7E3 Fab (abciximab) therapy. *Circulation* 1997;95:809–13.

Boggio LN, Green, D. Acquired hemophilia. *Rev Clin Exp Hematol* 2001;5:389–404.

Bounameaux H, Perneger T. Fondaparinux: a new synthetic pentasaccharide for thrombosis prevention. *Lancet* 2002;359:1710–11.

Caprie Steering Committee. A randomized, blinded trial of clopidogrel versus aspirin in patients at risk of ischaemic events (CAPRIE). *Lancet* 1996;348:1329–39.

Cure Investigators. Effects of clopidogrel in addition to aspirin in patients with acute coronary syndromes without ST-elevation. *N Engl J Med* 2001;345:494–502.

Feinstein DI, Green D, Federici AB, Goodnight SH Jr. Diagnosis and management of patients with spontaneously acquired inhibitors of coagulation. In: *American Society of Hematology Education Book*. Washington DC: American Society of Hematology, 1999:192–208.

Fennerty A, Campbell IA, Routledge PA. Anticoagulants in venous thromboembolism. *BMJ* 1988;297:1285–8.

Fitzmaurice DA, Machin SJ. Recommendations for patients undertaking self management of oral anticoagulation. *BMJ* 2001;323:985–9.

Fugh-Berman A. Herb–drug interactions. *Lancet* 2000;355:134–8.

Garcia Rodriguez LA, Jick H. Risk of upper gastrointestinal bleeding and perforation associated with individual non-steroidal anti-inflammatory drugs. *Lancet* 1994;343:769–72.

Greaves M, Cohen H, MacHin SJ et al. Guidelines on the investigation and management of the antiphospholipid syndrome. *Br J Haematol* 2000;109:704–15.

Guidelines on oral anticoagulation: third edition. *Br J Haematol* 1998;101:374–87.

Gurwitz JH, Gore JM, Goldberg RJ et al. Risk for intracranial hemorrhage after tissue plasminogen activator treatment for acute myocardial infarction. *Ann Intern Med* 1998;129:597–604.

Hylek EM, Chang YC, Skates SJ et al. Prospective study of the outcomes of ambulatory patients with excessive warfarin anticoagulation. *Arch Intern Med* 2000;160:1612–17.

Isles C, Norrie J, Paterson J, Ritchie L. Risk of major gastrointestinal bleeding with aspirin. *Lancet* 1999;353:148–50.

Landefeld CS, Beyth RJ. Anticoagulant-related bleeding: clinical epidemiology, prediction, and prevention. *Am J Med* 1993; 95:315–28.

Landefeld CS, McGuire E, Rosenblatt MW. A bleeding risk index for estimating the probability of major bleeding in hospitalized patients starting anticoagulant therapy. *Am J Med* 1990;89:569–78.

Levine MN, Raskob G, Landefeld S, Kearon C. Hemorrhagic complications of anticoagulant treatment. *Chest* 2001;119:108–21S.

Macik BG, Wang P. Management of warfarin-induced bleeding. In: Alving BM, ed. *Blood Components and Pharmacologic Agents in the Treatment of Congenital and Acquired Bleeding Disorders.* Bethesda, MD: AABB Press, 2000: 215–39.

Maggioni AP, Franzosi MG, Santoro E et al. The risk of stroke in patients with acute myocardial infarction after thrombolytic and antithrombotic treament (Gissi-2). *N Engl J Med* 1992;327:1–6.

Ortel TL. Clinical and laboratory manifestations of anti-factor V antibodies. *J Lab Clin Med* 1999; 133:326–34.

Sasahara AA, St Martin CC, Henkin J, Barker WM. Approach to the patient with venous thromboembolism. Treatment with thrombolytic agents. *Hematol Oncol Clin North Am* 1992;6:1141–59.

Sharis PJ, Cannon CP, Loscalzo J. The antiplatelet effects of ticlopidine and clopidogrel. *Ann Intern Med* 1998;129:394–405.

Topol EJ, Byzova TV, Plow EF. Platelet GpIIb-IIIa blockers. *Lancet* 1999;353:227–31.

Weitz JI, Leslie B, Ginsberg J. Soluble fibrin degradation products potentiate tissue plasminogen activator-induced fibrinogen proteolysis. *J Clin Invest* 1991; 87:1082–90.

Wells PS, Holbrook AM, Crowther NR, Hirsh J. Interactions of warfarin with drugs and food. *Ann Intern Med* 1994;121:676–83.

Useful addresses

For the clinician

Hemophilia and Thrombosis Research Society (HTRS)
Hemophilia Center
1415 Portland Ave #425
Rochester, NY 14621, USA
Tel: +1 585 922 5700
www.htrs.org/index.lasso

International Society on Thrombosis and Haemostasis
ISTH Headquarters, CB#7035
University of North Carolina at Chapel Hill School of Medicine
Chapel Hill
North Carolina 27599-7035
USA
Tel: +1 919 929 3807
Fax: +1 919 929 3935
www.med.unc.edu/isth/main.htm

British Committee for Standards in Haematology (BCSH): a subcommittee of the British Society for Haematology (for UK guidelines)
www.bcshguidelines.com

British Society for Haemostasis and Thrombosis
100 White Lion Street
London N1 9PF, UK
http:/med6.bham.ac.uk/bhst/

UK Haemophilia Doctors' Organisation
c/o Department of Haematology
Royal Infirmary, Oxford Road
Manchester M13 9WL, UK

For the patient

National Hemophilia Foundation
116 W 32nd Street, 11th Floor
New York, NY 10001, USA
Tel: +1 800 42 HANDI
www.hemophilia.org

**Platelet Disorder Support
Association**
P.O. Box 61533
Potomac, MD 20859, USA
Tel: +1 87 PLATELET
(+1 877 528 3538)
www.pdsa.org

**The Hereditary Hemorrhagic
Telangiectasia Foundation
International Website –**
Osler Weber Rendu
P.O. Box 329
Monkton, MD 21111, USA
Tel: +1 800 448 6389
www.hht.org/web/

World Federation of Hemophilia
1425 Rene Levesque Blvd. W.
Suite 1010
Montréal, Québec
H3G 1T7, Canada
Tel: +1 514 875 7944
wfh@wfh.org

The Haemophilia Society
Chesterfield House
385 Euston Road
London NW1 3AU, UK
Tel: +44 (0)20 7380 0600
Freephone: 0800 018 6068
info@haemophilia.org.uk
www.haemophilia.org.uk

ITP Support Association
'Synehurste'
Kimbolton Road
Bolnhurst MK44 2EW, UK
www.itpsupport.org.uk

Index

eptifibatide 115
erythropoietin 85
estrogen 25
eyes, hemorrhage 17, 24, 38

factor II (prothrombin) 10, 74, 79, 96
factor V
autoantibodies to 98–9
deficiency 61, 74, 80, 81, 96
hemostasis 10, 12
factor VII
deficiency 72–3, 74, 76, 79, 81, 96
hemostasis 10, 11, 87
recombinant 33, 100, 110
factor VIII
antibodies to 59, 61, 98, 109–10
hemophilia A see hemophilia A & B
hemostasis 11, 12, 87
liver disorders/DIC 80, 81
raised 80, 105
vWD 50–1, 63, 65, 66, 68
factor IX
hemophilia B see hemophilia A & B
hemostasis 10
liver disorders 79
factor X
deficiency 29, 73–4, 79, 96
hemostasis 10, 11, 12, 87
inhibition by heparin 116
factor XI
deficiency (hemophilia C) 70–2, 76, 96
hemostasis 10, 11
factor XII 11, 20, 50, 96
factor XIII 10–11, 17, 75
family histories 16, 59–60, 70
fetal death 91, 103, 107

fibrin 7, 10
see also fibrinolysis
fibrin degradation products (FDPs) 13, 19, 105
fibrinogen
deficiency 33, 74–5, 76, 79
DIC 104, 105–6
hemostasis 9, 11
liver disorders 79, 81
pregnancy 87, 90
screening tests 19, 20
thrombolytic agents 123
fibrinolysis
DIC 82, 104, 105
hemostasis 7, 12–14, 87
inhibitors 13–14, 24–5, 48–50, 52, 68
liver disorders 79–80
folate 80
fondaparinux (pentasaccharide) 116, 117
full blood count 18–19, 35, 42

gastrointestinal bleeding 15, 24, 48, 82, 114, 115
Glanzmann thrombasthenia 32, 33
glycoproteins, platelet membrane 9, 32, 44, 45, 115
gold 43
gray platelet syndrome 33

HELLP syndrome 41, 89
hemarthroses 15, 17, 55–6, 72
hematocrit 85, 97
hematomas 15, 56, 58, 91, 117
hemolytic–uremic syndrome 41
hemophilia A & B 61
acquired 109–10
clinical features 17, 55–8, 96, 109

hemophilia A & B
continued
combined deficiencies 61, 74
epidemiology 53
female carriers 53, 55, 59–60
molecular genetics 16, 53–5
surgery 55, 58, 98
treatment 49–51, 58–9, 60–1, 110
hemophilia C 70–2, 76, 96
hemostasis, normal 7–14, 87
hemostasis, abnormal
laboratory tests 18–21, 35, 94–7
medical history 15–17, 21, 93
physical examination 17–18, 93
severity index 113
Henoch–Schönlein purpura 26–7, 30
heparin 17, 82, 95–6, 99–100, 106, 107, 116–18
heparin-induced thrombocytopenia (HIT) 41, 44, 98, 117–18
hepatitis
cause of coagulation disorders 27–8, 78–80, 81–2
infected clotting factor concentrates 60–1, 68–9
herbal remedies 35, 43, 94, 120–1
hereditary hemorrhagic telangiectasia (HHT) 17, 23–5
Hermansky–Pudlak syndrome 33
HIV 35, 43, 60
hydroxyurea 34
hypertension
portal 78
in pregnancy 89, 91
hypotension 103

surgery *continued*
  intraoperative bleeding
  16, 97–8, 100
  postoperative bleeding
  16, 98–9
  thrombocytopenia 36,
  50, 98

tamoxifen 25
telangiectasia 17, 18, 23–5
thrombin
  DIC 103–4
  hemostasis 8, 10–11,
  14
  inhibitors 11–12, 122–3,
  125
thrombin activatable
  fibrinolytic inhibitor
  (TAFI) 13–14
thrombocythemia 34
thrombocytopenia
  causes 35–6, 41–5, 98
  definition 34
  diagnosis 17, 34–5,
  37–9, 42
  DIC 82, 105
  dilutional 92, 97
  heparin-induced 41, 44,
  98, 117–18
  ITP 36–41, 42–3, 46,
  87–8, 92
  liver disorders 80, 82
  neonatal 43, 88–9
  perioperative 36, 97, 98
  in pregnancy 41–3, 87,
  92

thrombocytopenia
  continued
  treatment 39–41, 42–3,
  45–6, 50
  vWD 65, 67
thrombolytic agents
  123–5
thrombomodulin 8, 12
thrombopoietin 43–4, 80
thrombosis 12, 72, 75, 84,
  87, 112, 118
thrombotic
  microangiopathies 37, 41
thrombotic
  thrombocytopenic
  purpura (TTP) 41, 43,
  63
ticlopidine 43, 115
tirofiban 115
tissue factor (TF) 8, 10,
  102, 103–4
tissue factor pathway
  inhibitor 12
tissue plasminogen
  activator (tPA) 13, 104,
  124–5
tranexamic acid 25,
  48–50, 52, 68
transforming growth
  factor β (TGFβ) 23
transfusions
  clotting factors 58–9,
  60–1, 67–9, 72, 73, 74,
  75, 82
  platelets 33, 45–6, 82,
  106, 115

transfusions *continued*
  post-transfusion purpura
  44
  red cells 85, 92
Turner's sign 17

uremia 82–6
urinary tract 49
urokinase 49, 124–5

valproic acid 33–4
vasopressin *see*
  desmopressin
vincristine 41
vitamin C 25–6
vitamin K
  deficiency 74, 79, 82,
  96–7
  warfarin 118, 120
von Willebrand's disease
  (vWD) 69
  clinical features 63–4
  diagnosis 15, 64–6
  treatment 50–1, 66–9
von Willebrand factor
  (vWF)
  hemostasis 7–8, 9, 63,
  64, 87
  renal failure 84
  treatment of vWD 67–9

warfarin 73, 118–22, 125
Wiskott–Aldrich
  syndrome 33, 35

ximelagatran 123

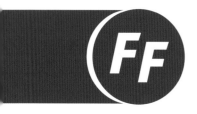

FAST FACTS

An outstandingly successful independent medical handbook series

Over one million copies sold

- Written by world experts
- Concise and practical
- Up-to-date
- Well structured for ease of reading and reference
- Copiously illustrated with useful photographs, diagrams and charts

Our aim for *Fast Facts* remains the same as ever: **to be the world's most respected medical handbook series**. Feedback on how to make individual titles even more useful is always welcome (feedback@fastfacts.com).

Some of the *Fast Facts* titles available

Allergic Rhinitis

Benign Gynecological Disease (second edition)

Benign Prostatic Hyperplasia (fourth edition)

Bladder Cancer

Breast Cancer (second edition)

Celiac Disease

Colorectal Cancer (second edition)

Contraception

Dementia

Depression

Diseases of the Testis

Disorders of the Hair and Scalp

Dyspepsia (second edition)

Endometriosis (second edition)

Epilepsy (second edition)

Erectile Dysfunction (third edition)

Gynecological Oncology

Headaches (second edition)

HIV in Obstetrics and Gynecology

Hyperlipidemia (second edition)

Hypertension (second edition)

Inflammatory Bowel Disease

Irritable Bowel Syndrome (second edition)

Menopause

Minor Surgery

Multiple Sclerosis

Osteoporosis (third edition)

Prostate-Specific Antigen (second edition)

Psoriasis

Respiratory Tract Infection (second edition)

Rheumatoid Arthritis

Schizophrenia (second edition)

Sexually Transmitted Infections

Soft Tissue Rheumatology

Superficial Fungal Infections

Travel Medicine

Urinary Continence (second edition)

Urinary Stones

For a complete list of books and more information on individual titles, to order online or to find regional distributors, please go to

www.fastfacts.com

For telephone orders, please call +44 (0)1752 202301 (UK & Europe) or 1 800 538 1287 (North America, toll free)

Forthcoming and recently published titles

Fast Facts – Benign Prostatic
Hyperplasia (fifth edition)
by Roger S Kirby, London, UK, and
John D McConnell, Texas, USA

Fast Facts – Parkinson's Disease
by Christopher G Clough, London, UK,
K Ray Chaudhuri, London, UK, and
Kapil D Sethi, Georgia, USA

Fast Facts – Smoking Cessation
by Robert West, London, UK, and
Saul Shiffman, Pittsburgh, USA

Fast Facts – Eczema and
Contact Dermatitis
by John Berth-Jones, Warwickshire, UK,
Eunice Tan, Norfolk, UK, and
Howard Maibach, San Francisco, USA

Fast Facts – Infant Nutrition
by Alan Lucas, London, UK,
and Stanley Zlotkin,
Toronto, Canada

Fast Facts – Acne
by Alison M Layton, Yorkshire, UK,
Diane Thiboutot, Pennsylvania, USA, and
Vincenzo Bettoli, Ferrara, Italy

Fast Facts – Anxiety, Panic and Phobias
(second edition)
by Malcolm H Lader, London, UK, and
Thomas W Uhde, Detroit, USA

Fast Facts – Chronic Obstructive
Pulmonary Disease
by William MacNee, Edinburgh, UK, and
Stephen I Rennard, Nebraska, USA

Fast Facts – Sexual Dysfunction
by S Michael Plaut, Baltimore, USA,
Alessandra Graziottin, Milan, Italy, and
Jeremy PW Heaton, Kingston, Canada

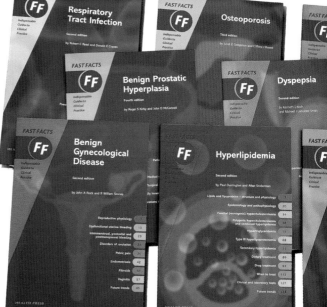

Health Press
medical publishing
at its best